S0-BWT-132

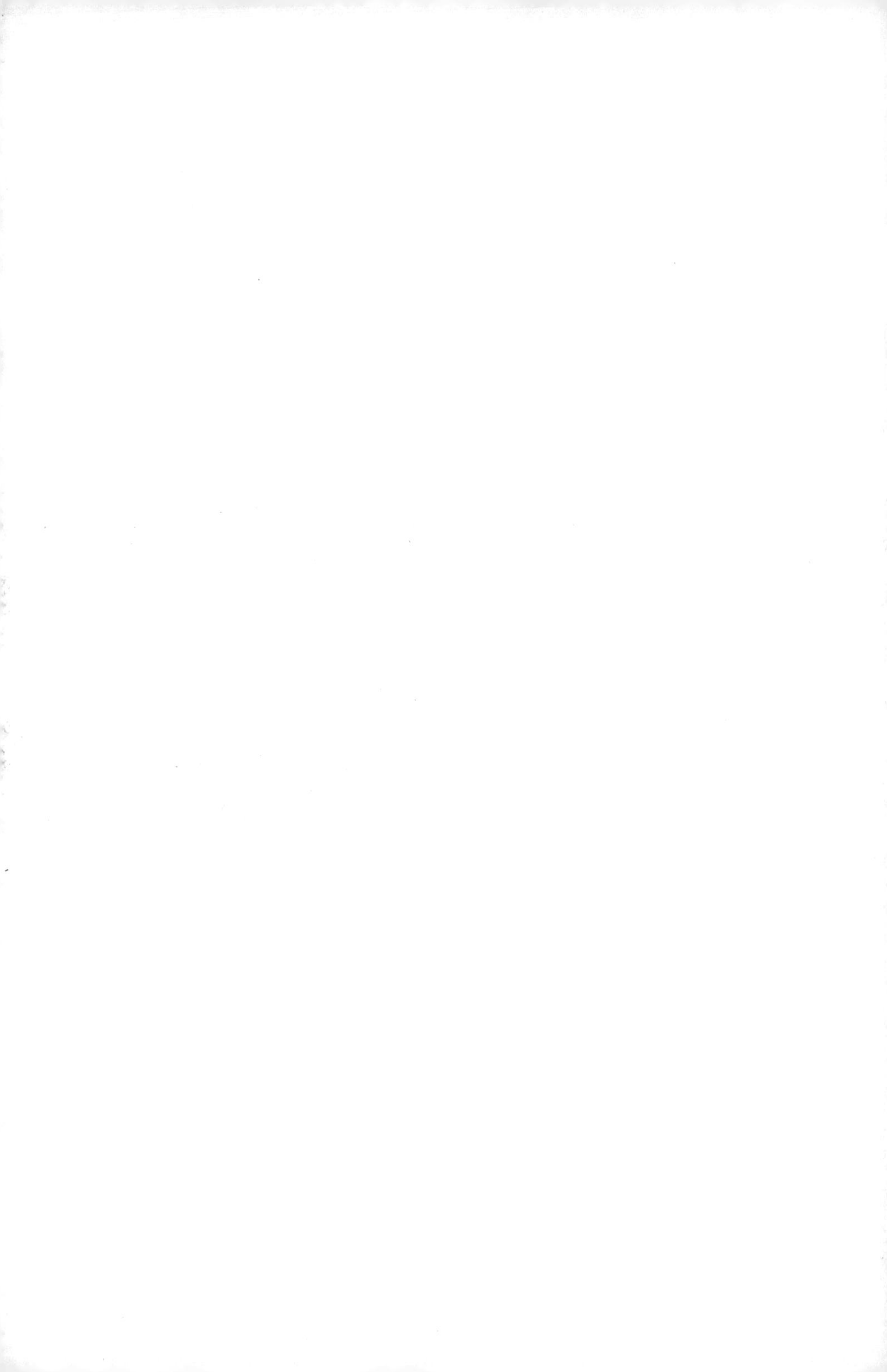

Child Language Disability: Implications in an Educational Setting

Multilingual Matters

Bilingual Children: From Birth to Teens
GEORGE SAUNDERS
Bilingualism: Basic Principles
HUGO BAETENS BEARDSMORE
Bilingualism or Not: The Education of Minorities
TOVE SKUTNABB-KANGAS
Cultural Studies in Foreign Language Education
MICHAEL BYRAM
Every Child's Language
(Open University Pack)
Key Issues in Bilingualism and Bilingual Education
COLIN BAKER
Language Acquisition of a Bilingual Child
ALVINO FANTINI
Language in a Black Community
VIV EDWARDS
Marriage Across Frontiers
A. BARBARA
Minority Education: From Shame to Struggle
T. SKUTNABB-KANGAS and J. CUMMINS (eds.)
Minority Education and Ethnic Survival
MICHAEL BYRAM
The Open Door
FINBARRE FITZPATRICK
Oral Language Across the Curriculum
DAVID CORSON
Raising Children Bilingually: The Pre-school Years
LENORE ARNBERG
Sign and School
JIM KYLE (ed.)
Story as Vehicle
EDIE GARVIE
Young Children in China
R. LILJESTRÖM *et al.*

Child Language Disability:
Implications in an Educational Setting

Edited by

Kay Mogford and Jane Sadler

MULTILINGUAL MATTERS LTD
Clevedon · Philadelphia

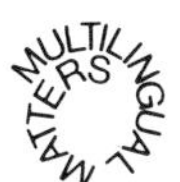

Library of Congress Cataloging in Publication Data
Child language disability
Bibliography: p.
Includes index.
1. Learning disabled children — Education — Language arts. 2. Language disorders in children. I. Mogford, Kay. II. Sadler, Jane.
LC4704.85.C48 1989 371.9′044 89-3102

British Library Cataloging in Publication Data

Child language disability: implications in an educational setting.
1. Language disordered children. Remedial education
I. Mogford, Kay, *1945–*
II. Sadler, Jane
371.91′4

ISBN 1-85359-052-5
ISBN 1-85359-051-7 Pbk

Multilingual Matters Ltd
Bank House, 8a Hill Road & 242 Cherry Street
Clevedon, Avon BS21 7HH Philadelphia, Pa 19106-1906
England USA

Cover design by Jussi Nurmi.
Index compiled by Meg Davies (Society of Indexers).
Typeset by SuttonPrint, Paignton.
Printed and bound in Great Britain by Short Run Press, Exeter.

Contents

Preface vii

Notes on Contributors ix

Specific Language Impairment — A Specific or Pervasive Developmental Disorder?
Kay Mogford 1

1 Language Development in the School Years — What Can Go Wrong?
Corinne Haynes 8

2 Relationship Between Spoken and Written Language Disorders
Joy Stackhouse 22

3 The Speech and Language Problems Screening-Test (SLPS)
Joanne Corcoran 31

4 Screening and Intervention with Children with Speech and Language Difficulties in Mainstream Schools
Ann Locke 40

5 Staged Assessment in Literacy: Implications for Language Problems in Secondary Schools
Michael Beveridge 52

6 Structuring the Curriculum in a Language Unit
Ella Hutt 65

7 Patterns of Mathematical Learning Associated with Language Disorder
Chris Donlan 76

8 The Parents' Role in Supporting Children in Education
Richard Da Costa 83

9 The Work of the Association For All Speech Impaired Children
Moira Noble 90

Index 99

Preface

On 23 April 1988 a conference was held on *Children with Language Difficulties: Implications in an Educational Setting,* organised by the Department of Speech of the University of Newcastle upon Tyne in association with Sunderland Education Authority.

An attendance of over 400 participants, including teachers from mainstream and special schools, support services and language units, speech therapists, educational psychologists and parents of language disordered children, testifies to the lack of easily available knowledge and expertise to help provide more effectively for the special educational needs of children with language handicaps.

It is hoped that the papers included in this volume, expanded to include material necessarily excluded in a 40 minute oral presentation, will not only give conference participants a more permanent record for reflective reading but also provide access to the topics for a much wider audience of readers.

Opportunities for in-service training for professionals on language handicaps appear to have been mainly concentrated in the south of England. This causes an additional drain on the limited time and financial resources available to those from the north who wish to keep abreast of developments in research and practice in this field.

We have been fortunate here in the Department of Speech at the University of Newcastle upon Tyne to be able to partially remedy this with the opening in September 1987 of a two-year part-time Diploma of Advanced Educational Studies course for experienced teachers on Child Language and Language Disability. In our efforts to bring to these teachers the most recent developments in this field, we were aware of the limited and modest literature available, particularly regarding the practical aspects of teaching. At the same time we knew of various experienced practitioners and research workers around the country who were pioneering new approaches and acquiring further expertise in solving the problems of professionals concerned with the educational difficulties of children with speech and language impairments.

We decided therefore to invite these colleagues to take part in a day conference and share their insights with local teachers, speech therapists and educational psychologists and to open the forum to those from further afield who felt they could benefit from the experience. It was hoped that such an occasion could provide an excellent opportunity not only to develop an awareness of the complexity and extent of this field in those professionals less versed in the subject but also to emphasise to as large and varied an audience as possible, the desirability and feasibility of a team approach to language remediation.

This book should not be considered as giving comprehensive coverage to the topic, but we hope it will provide useful information on recent developments and be a source of ideas for teachers and speech therapists who are working in a variety of educational settings with children of different ages and degrees of language handicap.

Finally we would like to take this opportunity to express our sincere thanks to all those who have helped us at various stages of this initiative: Mike Vening and Eileen Richardson, Special Educational Needs, Sunderland Education Authority for their assistance on the organising committee; Trevor Moon of the Tyneside Regional Group, Richard Da Costa and Moira Noble from the Headquarters of the Association For All Speech Impaired Children (AFASIC) who in addition to their moral support and encouragement made their contribution at the conference free of charge; Ann Stals and Pauline List for their secretarial assistance; Roy Bevan and Mike Grover, without whom this volume would not have been published.

Kay Mogford
Jane Sadler

Newcastle upon Tyne
August 1988

Notes on contributors

Kay Mogford is a speech therapist and developmental psychologist. As a lecturer in the Department of Speech at the University of Newcastle-upon-Tyne she teaches undergraduates who are training to be speech therapists and experienced teachers on the course in Child Language and Language Disability. Her research interests centre on the development of communication and related abilities in children with a range of developmental disorders affecting language development.

Corinne Haynes is Head Speech Therapist at Dawn House School for children with severe specific language disabilities where she has worked in close co-operation with teachers and other professionals. She has also carried out research in a number of areas related to the helping of children with specific language disabilities.

Joy Stackhouse is a speech therapist and psychologist who has specialised in research and professional practice in children's spoken and written language disorders. She is a Senior Lecturer in the School of Speech Therapy at Birmingham Polytechnic and an advisor for the College of Speech Therapists on developmental language disorders. At Birmingham she is currently helping to set up a distance learning course for teachers wishing to specialise in language disorders.

Joanne Corcoran is a research psychologist working in the School of Speech Pathology, Leicester Polytechnic. She is involved with two research projects, one aimed at devising and evaluating a speech and language screening test for children of six to ten years, the other aimed at developing a speech and language screen for use with nursery aged children.

Ann Locke is a speech therapist, teacher and educational psychologist. She is currently employed by Birmingham Education Department as Co-ordinator of Teaching Services for children with speech and language impairments. Her main responsibility is setting up services for these children in mainstream nursery, primary and secondary schools.

Michael Beveridge is a developmental and educational psychologist who currently teaches both undergraduates and experienced teachers at the University of Manchester. He previously lectured to speech therapists at Lancaster Polytechnic and was involved in research in mental handicap at the Hester Adrian Research Centre, Manchester University. His book, *Language Disability in Children* (with Gina Conti-Ramsden) was published in 1987 by the Open University Press. He is currently co-directing the Joint Matriculation Board's 'Staged Assessments in Literacy' project.

Ella Hutt draws on more than 20 years' experience teaching five to nine year old children with severe specific speech and language disorders in a small residential school. She is currently the project leader of the ICAN Curriculum Development and Resource Unit which aims to help staff of language units and schools whose children need a carefully structured curriculum.

Chris Donlan has taught language-impaired children in both 'specialised' and 'integrated' settings. He is currently Northern Region representative of the ICAN Curriculum Development and Resource Unit. He is researching mathematical learning in young children with language disorders and working with teachers and speech therapists on a curriculum study of mathematics in Language Units.

Richard Da Costa is the Chairman of AFASIC. He is the father of two boys with speech and language disorders who attend the Percy Hedley School in Newcastle which caters for the special needs of children with speech and language disabilities.

Moira Noble is the Associate Director for the Association For All Speech Impaired Children, with responsibility for Education and Press/Public Relations.

Specific language impairment — a specific or pervasive developmental disorder?

KAY MOGFORD

The educational implications of language difficulties cannot be adequately addressed unless the nature of those language difficulties are properly understood. In nearly all the papers included in this book, reference is made to the complex consequences of failure in language development for the lives and development of afflicted children and the implications for those involved in their care, whether as parent, teacher, speech therapist, psychologist or social worker. This paper provides a brief outline and discussion of the nature of language disability, as an introduction to this volume in which each other contributor discusses a different aspect of the disability, its identification and remediation.

Even five years ago, a discussion of developmental language difficulties would have been regarded as of marginal relevance to teachers in mainstream primary schools or even teachers in special education. Elizabeth Browning, former chairman of AFASIC, writing in March 1983, complains that 'failure in language development has been treated for so long with so much painful neglect'. She points out that in special education, while the needs of children with physical, sensory, or mental disabilities are always apparently recognised without argument, for the

> specifically speech and language disordered, cases have to be made, proved, fought and recognition and understanding won before anyone is prepared to even consider appropriate action to help the afflicted child.

It was encouraging then, in April 1988, when the conference organised by the Department of Speech, on the educational implications of specific language disability, was attended by over 400 participants, most of whom had a professional interest in providing for the needs of children with language difficulties in an educational context. This suggested an increase in concern for the educational needs of language-impaired children in the last few years. How can this recent rise in interest be explained?

Two reasons are worth examining briefly, both relating directly to the 1981 Education Act. Under this Act, the effort to classify and pigeon-hole children according to their primary disability before deciding on appropriate placement was replaced by the requirement to specify instead the special educational needs of each child. As this requirement is being implemented, it is becoming evident just how frequently the need to improve language use and understanding is identified as a special need irrespective of the child's primary disability. Many children who have differing disabilities share similar educational needs that originate in the slow development of language. This is in addition to those children, whose difficulties we will consider here, who have what is known as a specific language impairment. The term 'specific' is intended to convey that although the cause of this condition is unknown it is not the result of any other handicap. Until recently, when and if children with specific language impairment were recognised, educational provision was made for them, at the primary level, either in schools catering specially for those with developmental language disorders or in language units attached to mainstream schools. As a result, only a few specialised teachers were involved in this aspect of special education. Following implementation of the 1981 Act, their needs have been brought to the attention of a much larger number of teachers. Firstly, more children with less severe forms of disability are being recognised in mainstream schools and, secondly, children with more severe disorders are being integrated into mainstream classrooms (Sharron, 1988). As a result of both these developments, the size of the problem is also becoming clearer. Other contributors to this book, namely Locke and Corcoran, have a more detailed discussion of numbers of children with specific language disabilities. These numbers are little more than estimates that vary with the age of the population studied and the type of difficulties identified and there is some reason to believe that in the past the size of the problem has been underestimated (Enderby & Phillip, 1986). As the scale of the problem in educational terms is revealed, the inadequacy of our current ability to respond to these special needs in terms of human resources and understanding is also made more apparent.

A further reason for previous under-estimates of the numbers of children with specific language disabilities may have been the lack of recognition of the link between disorders of written and spoken language which is now established (Fundudis *et al,* 1979; Silva *et al,* 1983). It is only comparatively recently that the persistent though changing form of specific language impairment has been appreciated. Longitudinal studies have revealed how early problems with oral language have been associated with later difficulties in literacy (Fundudis *et al,* 1979; King *et al,* 1982; Silva *et al,* 1983; Aram *et al,* 1984).

Specific Language Impairment

If we consider evidence from a variety of circumstances in which children grow up we find that language is a surprisingly robust aspect of human development. It emerges in more or less adequate forms in some of the most apparently discouraging and unpromising circumstances (Mogford & Bishop, 1988). This makes it even more puzzling when children growing up in environments with few adverse circumstances experience difficulty in acquiring the language of their community with the facility of many apparently disadvantaged children, when they have no disability that would account for it. These are the children said to suffer from a specific language impairment. Reading about this topic is complicated because a variety of other terms have been used to refer to this condition, among the most common are developmental dysphasia and (developmental) language disorder. Language *disorder* is often distinguished from language *delay* though in the early stages of development the distinction is more theoretical than practical since the first manifestation of a disorder is a delay in language development. The distinction is made because children with a *delay* in language development may catch up with their peers in time, and/or with low level intervention. However it is not a simple matter to predict which children's difficulties will resolve with minimal intervention (Bishop & Edmundson, 1987a). However, children with a language disorder are thought to have a difficulty in the process of learning language which may not only delay but distort the pattern of language development. This implies that children with a language disorder need more intensive, long term intervention which is tailored to their individual requirements.

Children with a specific language impairment have none of the primary disabilities that would interfere with language development, such as deafness or mental handicap, yet their difficulties may be severe and persist even when they are given the best language learning conditions that we yet know how to provide. Following the terminology of the American Psychiatric Association, laid down in their Diagnostic and Statistical Manual (D.S.M. III — Revised, 1987), often regarded as the major reference for current terminology, these children are clearly classified as having a specific developmental disorder. This means that their condition is regarded as one in which only the function of language fails to develop while all other developmental areas are intact. This distinguishes the disorder from a general developmental delay on one hand and a pervasive developmental disorder on the other. A pervasive developmental disorder is one in which a core disturbance pervades many areas of development at the same time, and leads not so much to a delay but to a distortion in development, for example, as in autism. While there is no intention to challenge the classification of the D.S.M. III, the literal interpretation of the term 'specific' is misleading for this implies that only the area of language development is affected when, in reality, the effects of a failure in language acquisition are rarely, if ever, limited to this area of development. The effects of a failure in language development cannot help but distort the path of development to a degree. This is self-evident if we consider the role of language in cognitive and social development alone. In addition, failure in language development is often associated with developmental difficulties that cannot be seen entirely as the effects of this failure but related to the basic difficulty, for example motor and attentional difficulties. This view is not one arrived at through clinical experience alone but is based on studies published in the last decade (Silva *et al,* 1983; Bishop & Edmundson, 1987b). There is no intention to enter a further controversy over terminology but unless we attend to the complex developmental implications of developmental language disorders then our response in practical terms is likely to be misguided and inadequate.

It is suggested that a developmental language disorder is pervasive rather than specific, though the word pervasive is used in a rather broader sense than is intended in D.S.M. III. Language disorders can be considered pervasive in at least three ways.

Firstly, the effects of a language impairment pervade other aspects of development so that the normal balance and sequence is upset. This has implications for assessment as well as intervention. For example, as mentioned before, motor development is frequently found to be immature. Children with language disorders often appear to be clumsy and may have a poor body image. This means that if the nature of their difficulties is not understood, they may be expected to be competent in areas in which they in fact have difficulty. They may, on the other hand, develop a special facility in tasks relatively unaffected by their disability, for example, shape discrimination and completing form-boards. This may indicate greater potential for learning than they possess if assessed in this area alone. Some aspects of play, particularly imaginative play, may be slow to develop (Udwin & Yule, 1983; Terrell *et al,* 1984). Language disorder also reduces the opportunity for verbal interaction with other children and social skills are correspondingly slower to develop.

Secondly, a developmental language disorder can pervade several different aspects of language acquisition. Problems in oral expression may be noticed first: difficulties in developing a full range of speech sounds used in the language of the adult community, omission of grammatical words, the prolonged use of infant forms, excessive repetition, and hesitation or over rapid speech are obvious to a listener. However, difficulties are rarely confined to expressive language alone (Bishop, 1979). We may be less aware of a child's difficulties in understanding us. Failure to respond appropriately may instead be attributed to inattention, lack of co-operation or lack of intelligence. Alternatively some of a child's expressive difficulties may be attributed to a failure in the language learning environment. For example, knowledge of common words may appear to be very limited when in reality the child has difficulty in recalling words from memory when they are needed. Even when there has been some progress in these aspects of language, difficulties can persist: conversations can be strange and frustrating because the conventions of conversational exchange have not been mastered or because the child cannot infer a speaker's intentions accurately from what he says.

Thirdly, a developmental language disorder pervades many stages of development. Although the first evidence of a language disorder may be slowness to understand and/or speak in infancy, the pattern of ability and disability changes with development. With help and intervention in the pre-school years a child may still enter school with sufficient understanding and use of spoken language to cope in the early stages of primary education. However as the child approaches literacy the problems re-appear in learning to read and write (Fundudis *et al,* 1979; Silva *et al,* 1983).

Since the discovery of the condition was first made by medical practitioners in the last century, other disciplines and professions have been involved in the identification, management and remediation of specific language impairments. Each of these professions bring to this work their own systems of thought, philosophies and methods that are not always compatible. This is one reason for the variety of terminology. Inter-professional co-operation is not an easy task but is essential if children with this disabling problem are to be aided. Each contributor in this volume, is involved in some way, either directly or indirectly with trying to solve the problems of these children and their families. It is sometimes forgotten that a communication problem involves all those with whom the child needs to communicate as well as the child himself. The families of these children are in the front line. The papers that follow are offered as an attempt to share experience, insight and understanding with a wider audience. Each contribution has a slightly different perspective which derives from the particular role that the author plays. To help the reader we have included brief details about each contributor (see p. ix). As you will appreciate, in the area of practice we are still very much at the stage of individual resourcefulness and ingenuity. Time and energy can be saved if this experience is shared with those involved in a similar endeavour. We may be able to improve practice by reflecting critically on it and then developing and experimenting with the model that has been described. The following papers are offered as a stage in this process.

References

American Psychiatric Association, 1987, *Diagnostic and Statistical Manual of Mental Disorders.* 3rd edn revised. Washington D.C.: American Psychiatric Association.

Aram, D.M., Ekelman, B.L. and Nation, J.E. 1984, Preschoolers with language disorders; ten years later. *Journal of Speech and Hearing Research* 27, 234–244.

Bishop, D.V.M. 1979, Comprehension in developmental language disorders. *Developmental Medicine and Child Neurology* 21, 225–238.

Bishop, D.V.M. and Edmundson, A. 1987a, Language impaired 4-year-olds; distinguishing transient from persistent impairment. *Journal of Speech and Hearing Disorders* 52, 156–173.

— 1987b, Specific language impairment as a maturational lag; evidence from longitudinal data on language and motor development. *Developmental Medicine and Child Neurology* 29, 442–459.

Browning, E. 1983, Letter. *Bulletin of the College of Speech Therapists* March. No. 371.

Enderby, P. and Phillip, R. 1986, Speech and language handicap; toward knowing the size of the problem. *British Journal of Disorders of Communication* 21(2), 151–167.

Fundudis, T., Kolvin, I. and Garside, R. (eds) 1979, *Speech Retarded and Deaf Children; Their Psychological Development.* London: Academic Press.

King, R.R., Jones, C. and Lasky, E. 1982, In retrospect, a 15-year follow-up of speech-language disordered children. *Language, Speech and Hearing Services in Schools* 13, 24–32.

Mogford, K. and Bishop, D. 1988, Five questions about language acquisition considered in the light of exceptional circumstances. In D. Bishop and K. Mogford (eds) *Language Development in Exceptional Circumstances.* Edinburgh: Churchill Livingstone.

Sharron, H. 1988, Integration. Flourishing in a brand new environment. *Challenge* Summer. ICAN.

Silva, P.A., McGee, R. and Williams, S.M. 1983, Developmental language delay from 3 to 7 years and its significance for low intelligence and reading difficulties at age seven. *Developmental Medicine and Child Neurology* 25, 783–793.

TERRELL, B.Y., SCHWARTZ, R.C., PRELOCK, P.A. and MESSICK, C.K. 1984, Symbolic play in normal and language impaired children. *Journal of Speech and Hearing Research* 27, 424–429.

UDWIN, O. and YULE, W. 1983, Imaginative play in language disordered children. *British Journal of Disorders of Communication* 18(3), 197–206.

1 Language development in the school years — what can go wrong?

CORINNE HAYNES

We no longer believe with McNeill (1970) that language development is completed between the ages of 18 months and 5 years. It starts much earlier and goes on much longer, and is inextricably interwoven with every other aspect of child development. Language and learning during the school years form a fine balancing act which contributes to rich and fruitful development in nearly all children. For those vulnerable children with language difficulties however, the school years are the time when imbalance has devastating effects. This paper is concerned with the normal development of meaning, grammar, use of language and speech in school children, and the ramifications of breakdown in any area in communication and education.

Every year large numbers of five-year-olds enter school for the first time. They come with a wide variety of abilities. Some children will be bubbling with eagerness and enthusiasm, others will be more timid and withdrawn but almost all will be well able to express their needs, ask questions and make comments in suitably ordered strings of words. Twenty years ago it was assumed that these ably communicating children entered school with all the basic rules of the English language intact, and with only some expansion in depth still to take place. Since then, research in child language development has shown just what competence children bring to school at age five, and what linguistic discoveries they are going to make in the subsequent 10 to 12 years.

The average five-year-old in the reception class is a reasonably adequate and fluent communicator. He or she (henceforth 'he') can use complex sentences with generally mature syntax, although he may make occasional errors. He can vary the style of language; four-year-olds when talking to two-year-olds have been shown to use some of the features of the parent–child talk that is sometimes called 'motherese', such as shorter sentences, increased pitch range, and so on. He is intelligible, using a nearly complete system of the sounds of English. Any speech sounds that have not completely developed sound quite appropriate for a five-year-old child and do not impede communication. He has some useful discourse skills and can manipulate the environment quite well; he may be surprisingly subtle in gaining the desired goal.

The result of this apparent adequacy is that adults treat young children as rather more competent communicators than they are. Although adults probably adapt their language in some ways, use more content words and more repetitions and simplify their vocabulary, they also make a number of false assumptions about the children's language competence. This gap between actual and assumed linguistic ability probably creates the need for the child to hypothesise and experiment, and thus develop his skills. Adults and children actually bring rather different linguistic systems to their interactions and neither fully understands the system employed by the other. But whereas adults are somewhat fixed and inflexible in their language use, the child is an open and active language learner. Faced with some unknown vocabulary, or a complex bit of grammar, the child will use a set of strategies to make sense of it. After encountering numerous similar examples he will gradually develop an hypothesis about the underlying adult rules which govern this meaning or structure. He will then change his own strategies for generating language until the rules have become those of the adult language user. Normally this process will continue until adolescence but when this learning process fails, language impairment results.

Although language develops in different children at different rates and with personal idiosyncrasies, the course of language development in the school years is common to all children, and is linked to non-linguistic advances. This is good evidence, if we needed it, that language is just one thread in the intricately woven cloth of child development, where also are woven cognitive, perceptual, motor and social skills.

To discuss language development in an isolated way is rather like taking a child to the growth clinic and discussing with the paediatrician how his left leg is growing. Just as growth of the left leg only means something in relation to the whole and is only the focus of interest if it is growing faster or slower than the rest of the body, language does not develop in isolation from cognitive and social development. Nor do things go wrong with language development in a contained way; problems proliferate and intertwine affecting all other areas of development.

There are three types of children with language-learning difficulties that the teacher needs to watch for. The child with:

(1) *Problems resulting from non-specific factors.*
Excluding the major language disabling conditions such as autism, profound deafness and mental handicap, there are a number of lesser handicapping conditions which will affect language in school:
a conductive hearing loss (this usually results from an accumulation of fluid in the middle ear that reduces the conduction of sound to the inner ear, producing a mild and fluctuating hearing loss which may not be apparent after one testing),
physical or sensory disabilities,
adverse environmental factors,
emotional deprivation,
personality difficulties.
Almost anything that goes wrong with any aspect of the child's development will subsequently affect language development. Therefore the first course of action with any child showing language difficulties in school is a full investigation of his physical, mental and emotional situation. This should be as soon after school entry as possible. These are vital years.

(2) *A 'hidden' specific difficulty.*
Such a child has always had an underlying language deficit, but because of good compensatory skills on his part, perhaps coupled with limited demands in his environment and parents who go more than halfway to meet his needs, this may not become apparent until entering school. Here he fails to develop the more cognitively demanding and subtle skills which will enable him to participate in classroom activities, particularly literacy skills. Indeed, it can happen that such a child gets by in infant school, and only the increasingly verbal requirements of junior school reveal his difficulties.

(3) *Specific developmental language disorder.*
This child's difficulties have always been apparent. As the gap between chronological age and language ability widens, he becomes increasingly unable to cope. The language problems become compounded by learning difficulties and social and emotional problems.

All of these children deserve skilled specific help. The child in the third category may eventually receive special provision although this may not occur until he has been struggling unaided, for some time, in a mainstream class. However, children in the first two categories may well not get any special help other than that provided by a concerned classroom teacher.

The teacher can provide basic support to a child falling into any of these categories in three ways:

(1) by using less language-dependent methods in teaching skills (e.g. continuing the use of concrete apparatus for number work)
(2) by teaching strategies for learning which circumvent language-associated weaknesses (e.g. fostering the use of visual imaging to compensate for poor short term auditory verbal memory)
(3) by gaining better understanding of the child's difficulties within the framework of normal and abnormal language development (e.g. the use of language profiling, such as described in Crystal, 1982).

For the non-specialist teacher in a mainstream class, it is probably a better use of time and expertise if a speech therapist can be found to co-operate in any language profiling. However, as the teacher is the person who interacts with a child for a large part of each day, he or she needs to have some knowledge of the various areas of language — semantics, grammar, phonology and pragmatics and the interrelation between these skills — to have reasonable expectations of development, and to be able to pinpoint problems.

I want to describe briefly and in non-technical terms what these aspects of language are, and how they interrelate.

Semantics

The area we can take as basic to communication is meaning. Without meaning to convey or understand, there would be no communication. The study of meaning is called semantics and has three components:

(1) the meaning of words, that is the acquisition of concepts;
(2) the relationship of words to each other, whether in the same semantic field (e.g. gold, silver, tin, lead) or in some sort of hierarchical relationship (e.g. flora, plant, vegetable, tuber, potato), or in relationships such as opposition (hot, cold);
(3) the role words play to express meaning in sentences, indicating, for example, time, location, actor, or goal. These are different from grammatical roles. For example in the sentence, 'Maggie kissed the baby', grammatically, 'Maggie' is subject, semantically 'Maggie' is actor. In the sentence, 'The baby was annoyed', grammatically, 'the

baby' is now the subject; but semantically, 'the baby' is experiencer rather than actor.

Grammar

Grammar is closely related to semantics. It consists of:

(1) syntax, the rules that describe the possible combinations of words in sentences and phrases;
(2) morphology, changes to the word itself that indicate different grammatical roles, such as plurals, verb tenses.

Speech

There are two things to consider here, only the first of which is considered to be a level of language:

(1) phonology, this describes the way the speech sounds of any language are organised so that the contrasts between sounds alter meaning, e.g. 'male' and 'pale'; 'lie' and 'light'. Children with language difficulties frequently have phonological problems, and these are essentially problems with a linguistic system rather than a problem of motor co-ordination.
(2) articulation, this is included to complete the picture of speech production, although it is independent of language and refers to the physical ability to produce speech sounds; e.g. a child suffering from cerebral palsy, or cleft palate usually has an articulation problem although such a child may or may not have an additional language (i.e. phonological) problem. Equally a child with a specific phonological difficulty may, or may not, have an accompanying articulation problem.

Pragmatics

Finally, we have language in relation to its use in social context, i.e. pragmatics. This is the most recent area to come under close linguistic scrutiny, and there is no clear agreement as to its boundaries or component parts, or even whether it is properly part of language study. For a teacher interested in a child's use of language in the classroom, it could be helpful to consider:

(1) his verbal control of the environment; satisfaction of needs, requesting,

rejecting, denying, precipitating action in others, establishing roles and pecking orders;

(2) self fulfilment; self expression, expressing moods and emotions, giving information, getting information, learning;

(3) discourse — rules which govern conversation shared between two or more people, styles of address.

Semantics, grammar, phonology and pragmatics are the levels of language that will be considered in the discussion of language problems. Language disorder does not necessarily involve all these linguistic levels simultaneously, but rarely involves only one, discretely. It is most common to find some degree of interaction between different linguistic levels, and also interaction with other aspects of development.

The simple model in Figure 1 demonstrates the kind of interaction of linguistic levels that I have observed in language disordered children. (This is not a theoretical model, nor does it attempt to measure cause and effect, it is merely a schematic representation of clinical observations.) The direction of effect is upwards. Thus phonological problems can exist independently, and may not affect other aspects of language. They may sometimes affect pragmatics (the only area which is partially above phonology on the model). In contrast to that, a problem with semantics always affects other language functions, either grammar and phonology, or pragmatics, or all three.

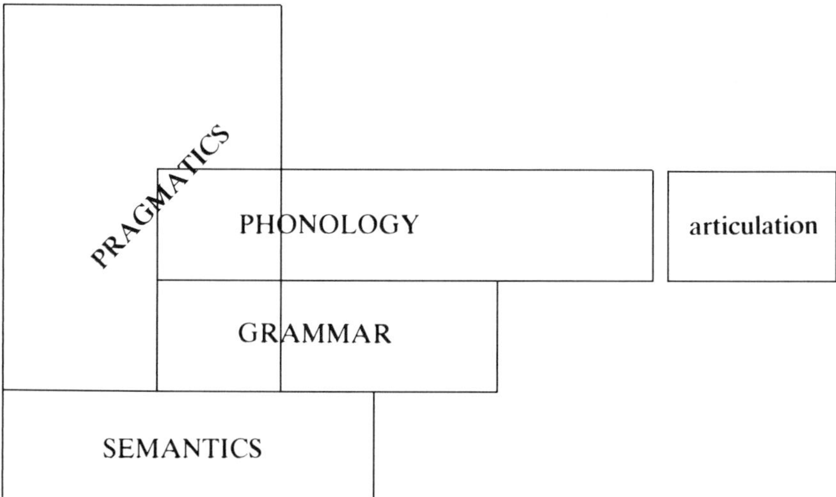

FIGURE 1 *Simple diagram of interactions of linguistic levels. Problems at lower levels affect those above them. Secondary effects are not shown.*

It should be quite obvious when a child is having some problems with language in the classroom if these occur mainly at the phonological or syntactic level. However semantic and pragmatic problems are a little harder to recognise. Although some minor problems, and others relating to lack of stimulation may diminish when a child enters school, for many children unfortunately, the verbal gap between them and their normal peers widens. The school curriculum at all ages relates to the expected normal development of skills and knowledge, and it is therefore essential to have some awareness of normal development in each area of language, when considering the special needs of the child with problems.

The normal development of phonology

Speech development is not complete at school entry, but is normally completed between 5 and 7 years of age, with the perfection of sounds such as 'r' and 'th' and some consonant clusters; words such as '*crisps*', '*str*ing', and polysyllabic words (e.g. hospital, elephant) may take some time to become accurate. These things are noticeable. More generally, and less well appreciated by adults is the relatively slow development of the full intonational system, which is considered an area of phonology. Cruttenden (1974) showed that 10-year-old football fans were not able to predict football results from the intonational patterns of sports reporters, whereas adults, not interested in sport, could guess before they heard the second team's score, whether a win, loss or draw was being announced. Cruttenden (1985) again found a range of intonational, or prosodic features as they are usually called, which were not interpreted correctly by 10-year-olds. For example, the 10-year-olds had difficulty understanding who gave Martha the orange in such sentences as 'John gave an apple to Sam, and then *he* gave an orange to Martha'. (According to the stress it might be John or Sam.) Appreciation of attitudinal intonation has also been shown to develop at this time, as in '*Mr* Smith's alright' (but as for Mrs Smith . . .). Intonation can also be used to indicate sarcasm, reservations and so forth. This sort of prosodic pointing, particularly use of stress, is very commonly used by adults, and often by teachers to pupils who have failed to grasp something the first time. If the pupils do eventually succeed it may not in fact be due to their appreciation of stress.

Abnormal development of phonology

Although phonological disability can occur without involving other aspects of spoken language, it is very likely to affect reading and writing and often co-occurs with some grammatical difficulties. Some language disordered children have a major problem with the establishment of a sound system. Typically these children use a small number of sounds to do the work of the 40 speech sounds used in English, not because they are unable to articulate them, but because they have not become an integral part of their internal language system. Although they may well be able to perceive gross differences, their perception of these sounds when used by others may be fuzzy. This has obvious social implications for intelligibility and results in impaired communication and frustration. Phonological disability has less obvious implications for semantics and syntax. Vocabulary acquisition must proceed at a slower rate, and grammatical inflections — many of which in English rely on a word-final /s/ — may not be produced. There are major educational implications for reading and spelling. The essential skills of sound analysis and sound-blending in words are not attained. It is this failure to develop an adequate internalised system and good internal representations of sounds, that particularly affects literacy skills, not, as is sometimes imagined, the inability to produce speech sounds.

Very little investigation of the development of intonation in language disordered children has been carried out. A small study at Dawn House School (Haynes & Tempest, 1984) into the perception of differences in pitch, length and rhythm found that the language disordered nine-year-olds had pitch and length awareness equivalent to a group of normal six-year-olds, and their rhythmic perception was deviant. About 20% of the Dawn House pupils also had mild to moderate abnormalities of production of intonation. The effect of this on pragmatics is clearly large, but the effects on acquiring vocabulary and learning the rules of English grammar, where rhythm is so important, may well be even larger.

Normal development of grammar

Most school entrants still need to sort out some irregular past tenses of verbs, including the present perfect, and irregular plural noun forms such as 'geese' and 'sheep'. The mistakes they still make tend to come from over-generalisation of regular rules — e.g. 'choosed', 'sheeps'.

Syntactically, quite a lot of development can be expected in the school years. Although five-year-olds come to school able to use subordination of clauses, the extent of its use, subtlety and complexity, develops enormously in the next three years. Embedded clauses develop such as 'the boy, *I saw you with yesterday,* wasn't your brother', as does cross reference using pronouns, '*Roger*'s cleverer than Sally, *he* always . . .'.

The acquisition of the passive voice is normally completed during the primary school period. Understanding of reversible passives (e.g. John was hit by Peter) is not expected before about 7;6, non-reversible passives may be understood using some sort of probable event strategy. In a sentence such as 'the sandwich was eaten by the boy', the child knows what is likely to happen in a real situation, and responds accordingly. Children make good use of probability and their knowledge of the world to sort out syntactic rules. Semantics seems to dominate syntax, thus of the two ways of negating the positive statement 'I think Joe will come' primary school children will use the more semantically meaningful, 'I think Joe won't come' rather than the more usual but rather (semantically) strange adult form, 'I don't think Joe will come'.

Abnormal development of grammar

For children with language problems, this is probably the area of most obvious difficulty, and is considerably affected by any associated problems with attention, perception, memory, rhythm, sequencing, organisation and motor ability.

Language disordered children often tend to string information bearing words together, omitting function words. They may not use any of the morphological inflections other than the verb ending '-ing', for a very long time. They have a particular problem with verbs and often with the pronoun system. They pause and struggle to produce the right structures, often making false starts and using empty words like 'thingy'. They sound like much younger children. Yet these are children of normal intelligence, able to conceptualise and form hypotheses (Kamhi *et al.*, 1984). They do derive rules from the language they hear, but in an idosyncratic manner. Their problems with attention are well documented.

Auditory short term memory is limited, so that processing capacity is much reduced, particularly for more complex structures. Adults have a variety of strategies for coping with the demands of language processing which are not available to a child with a language disorder. We use rhythm to chunk utterances — these children are dysrhythmic; we derive the meaning of complex sentences by extracting the meanings from a series of clauses, and saving them in mental shorthand — even if these children can extract the meaning of short clauses, they cannot organise and sequence them; we verbally rehearse to keep things in immediate memory while we work on them — these children have an inadequate immediate memory, an impaired sound system and slow articulation which hinders verbal rehearsal.

A child who cannot easily use the grammar of a sentence to work out its meaning, has to derive this in another way. This probably requires much more time, so he has little chance of untangling the implications of the message or drawing out subtle inferences. This has an inevitable effect on his classroom learning: no wonder he looks blank. A child who is given sentences in a reading book which, as in many of the early readers, are beyond his functional language level, cannot comprehend what he reads, and so gets little motivation to persevere with such an arduous task. Nor can such a child easily use internalised language to direct and organise his thinking and problem solving, or produce coherent, rational narrative accounts.

Normal development of semantics

In this bedrock of language, a great deal happens during the school years.

Five-year-olds have only a limited concept of many words, having incorporated some, but not all of the appropriate semantic features. Cruttenden (1979; 1985) says that, 'almost all children's words will, at one time or another, mean something different from the adult meaning'. Infants also have a lot to learn in the area of classifying and categorisation. They are about to be introduced to a wide variety of size, spatial and temporal concepts as part of number work. From the age of seven onwards, thinking will become increasingly abstract and symbolic in line with cognitive growth. From primary to secondary age, vocabulary just about doubles (Jenkins & Dixon, 1983). These are not just simple additions to their vocabulary but involve a restructuring of the field of word meanings, so that as a new concept is learned the relationships of word meanings to each other is adjusted. As the child develops the number of semantic roles possible in sentences (temporal, locative, etc.), is enlarged.

Here are a few examples, as a guideline to the way semantics develop and change. Further examples can be found in the bibliography listed at the end of this paper.

Spatial relationships. e.g. in front of, behind

(1) these are understood only in relationship to the child's own body;
(2) at the next stage, these terms develop meaning relative to objects with real fronts and backs;
(3) finally the concept of front and back of any object in relationship to itself is understood.

Left and right are even harder, and a child would normally be about nine years old before he could confidently use these terms in relation to others' bodies.

Connectives. Again one should expect stages of development, with some aspects of meaning being easier to grasp than others, for example the connective 'because' has three developmental stages:

(1) affective, e.g. 'Mary cried because Pat hurt her';
(2) causal, e.g. 'She stayed away because she was tired';
(3) logical, e.g. 'He's asleep because he's snoring.'

In general the greater the semantic complexity, the later these connectives are fully mastered, although they may be used appropriately in some contexts much earlier, giving adults a false expectation of the child's competence. Ages cited for full acquisition are:

'if' — six years;
'because' — seven years;
'unless' — nine years;
'although' — twelve years;
subtle distinctions of modifiers 'slightly', 'somewhat', 'quite' — teenage years.

Extended meanings. Some words have psychological referents in addition to concrete or perceptual meanings and the development of these is quite interesting. These are words such as 'sweet', 'bright', 'sharp'. Children under seven years of age use these terms in their concrete sense only, but between seven and eight, begin to use them in their psychological sense. However it is not until they are nine or ten that they understand the relationship between these two meanings.

Abnormal development of semantics

Semantic difficulties which become apparent in the child with a language disability are often an indication of a serious and long-term problem, involving (see Figure 1) many linguistic areas. Some possible interactions can be traced. Taking first word meaning; Susan Carey (1978) has described normal acquisition of words as having two paths, a conceptual path and a phonological path. When these converge, a child has learned a new word. A major problem for the language disordered child of course is the phonological path. The sound system deficiency means that this path is very slow and language disordered children need many more repetitions of a word before they begin to learn it. Normally at six years and over, children begin to code and store words phonically as they begin to acquire reading skills (Aitchison & Straf, 1981). For language disordered children their difficulties prevent this advance and they have to struggle on trying to store patterns of sound which have no visual correlate, and which they only perceive fuzzily in the first place.

In the area of semantics, that includes word categories and relationships, the gaps in concept acquisition make development patchy. Some areas are notoriously difficult for language disordered children (such as Time). Failure at one stage undermines the development of finer distinctions in meanings and poor organisational skills exacerbate the problem. Some children actively resist having to restructure their semantic fields, and cling to rigidly defined concepts.

The complex subordinators will not be understood or used properly, although adults increasingly expect this and use them more frequently in teaching situations. Indeed it is hard to envisage educational settings which do not make use of instructions such as, 'Do this after you have done that!' (temporal order differs from spoken order) and connectors like 'until', 'unless' and so on. Since a child's understanding of syntax may also be affected it cannot support semantics or vice versa, and there will be a vicious circle of confusion.

Normal development of pragmatics

It has been pointed out by Romaine (1984) that there is limited value in knowing the rules of language structure, unless you can use them to get things done. Very many features of appropriate and varied use of language have to be acquired by the school child, for example, more subtle techniques of persuasion or refusal or disapproval. Mention has been made of the development of some discourse features such as sentence connecting devices and cross reference in the discussion of semantics and syntax. Many others are developing at the pragmatic level; implied requests ('It's terribly hot in here' meaning 'please turn the fire down'.); inference ('Has John got a pencil sharpener?' 'Well, he borrowed mine yesterday'.); signalling conversational turns; topic repair or switching; awareness of shared or limited knowledge. As has been said, children use strategies for comprehending unknown grammatical structures, or non-verbal signals, based on their knowledge of what is probable, and their growing awareness of what is socially acceptable. The competence that they bring to school is altered partly by new experience, such as learning to read, and partly by social factors, such as peer group integration. From the narrow, shared and consistent world of family, they have to adapt to the much more varied world of the classroom and learn what knowledge is shared, and what must be explicated. They have to develop new language learning strategies suitable for a classroom where much (too much?) of the talk is teacher-initiated. Here most interactions are in groups, and children have to acquire a range of styles suitable for a variety of relationships and situations. They have to learn new ways of achieving their ends.

Abnormal development of pragmatics

The child with major pragmatic problems generally also has considerable difficulties with semantics, and in severe cases finds it extremely difficult to relate language in a meaningful way to the real world. Words seem almost too powerful; their meaning does not vary in context and cannot be subordinated to common sense. For these children words are masters, not tools. Such children are rare and need special help, but almost any language disordered child is likely to be somewhat disadvantaged in this area too and these pragmatic difficulties can be a source of adult complaint and misunderstanding. How often does one hear:

> 'He will interrupt when I'm dealing with another child'
> 'How can you do this if you don't look, or listen?'
> 'She is very rude'
> 'He always seems to miss the point'
> 'Sarcasm goes completely over her head'
> 'Wait for your turn'
> 'Why don't you do what you're told?'

These complaints may well result from pragmatic difficulties, but they are often perceived as wilful misbehaviour and can hinder the good teacher–pupil relationship necessary to promote learning. All the problems discussed with intonation, attention, short term memory, auditory perception, motor skills, semantics and syntax contribute to the problem here, and the ramifications of these difficulties have profound educational and social effects.

Conclusion

Language acquisition continues at least until adolescence. Children with language problems are likely to have their difficulties exacerbated by the increasing linguistic and cognitive demands of school life. Although problems can originate at different linguistic levels, the effects are broad, interactive and complex. An awareness of normal and abnormal language development during school years can help teachers to gain insight into particular problems, and provide a basis for remedial teaching.

Bibliography

AITCHISON, J. and STRAF, M. 1981, Lexical storage and retrieval: a developing skill? *Linguistics* 19 (7/8), 751–95.

CAREY, S. 1978, The child as word learner. In M. HALLE, K. BRESNAN and J. MILLER (eds) *Linguistic Theory and Psychological Reality*. Cambridge, MA: M.I.T. Press.

CRUTTENDEN, A. 1974, An experiment involving comprehension of intonation in children from 7 to 10. *Journal of Child Language* 1 (2), 221–32.

— 1979, *Language in Infancy and Childhood*. Manchester: Manchester University Press.

— 1985, Intonation comprehension in ten-year-olds. *Journal of Child Language* 12(3), 643–61.

CRYSTAL, D. 1976, *Child Language, Learning and Linguistics*. London: Edward Arnold.

— 1982, *Profiling Linguistic Disability*. London: Edward Arnold.

DONALDSON, M. 1978, *Children's Minds*. London: Fontana.

DURKIN, K. 1986, *Language Development in the School Years*. London: Croom Helm.

ELLIOT, A. 1981, *Child Language*. Cambridge: Cambridge University Press.

FLETCHER, P. and GARMAN, M. 1986, *Language Acquisition: Studies in First Language Development*. Second Edn. Cambridge: Cambridge University Press.

HARRIS, M. and COLTHEART, M. 1986, *Language Processing in Children and Adults*. London: Routledge & Kegan Paul.

HAYNES, C. and TEMPEST, B. 1984, Investigating the perception of prosodic features in language disordered children. Paper presented at the Child Language Seminar. Nottingham University.

JENKINS, J.R. and DIXON, R. 1983, Vocabulary learning. *Contemporary Educational Psychology* 8, 237–60.

KAMHI, A., CATTS, H., KOENIG, L. and LEWIS, B. 1984, Hypothesis testing and non-linguistic symbolic activity in language impaired children. *Journal of Speech and Hearing Disorders* 49(2), 169–76.

MCNEILL, D. 1970, *The Acquisition of Language*. London: Harper and Row.

ROMAINE, S. 1984, *The Language of Children and Adolescents*. Oxford: Blackwell.

WEBSTER, A. and MCCONNELL, C. 1987, *Children with Speech and Language Difficulties*. London: Cassell Educational.

WELLS, G. 1987, *The Meaning Makers: Children Learning Language and Using Language to Learn*. London: Hodder & Stoughton.

YULE, W. and RUTTER, M. 1987, *Language Development and Disorders*. London: MacKeith Press.

2 Relationship between spoken and written language disorders

JOY STACKHOUSE

Before learning to read and spell children have already established a psycholinguistic system to deal with spoken language. It is therefore not surprising that an intact facility for speech and language development appears to be a necessary prerequisite for satisfactory reading and spelling development. Evidence of a general relationship between speech and reading problems has been collected from a variety of sources. Perhaps the most well known is the Isle of Wight study carried out by Rutter & Yule (1973). In this study a variety of tests were administered to the nine-year-old population on the Isle of Wight. It was found that those children who had reading problems were characterised by earlier linguistic difficulties. Furthermore, within this reading-disabled group, generally backward readers could be differentiated from children with specific reading retardation. As in verbal language disorders these specific difficulties were more common in boys and often ran in the family. Similarly, in Edinburgh, Ingram *et al.* (1970) followed up a large group of children who had received speech therapy, to find that the majority of these were having reading difficulties. Finally, clinicians and teachers have often commented on the articulatory difficulties (Miles, 1982) or 'unclear speech' found in dyslexic children who are not identified as speech disordered or receiving any speech therapy.

Although a correlation between reading and speech difficulties has been demonstrated, few studies have examined the nature of the reading and spelling difficulties in children with different forms of speech handicap. To investigate the possibility that certain speech disordered groups may be more vulnerable than others to specific reading and spelling difficulties Stackhouse (1982) compared two groups of speech disordered children with normal controls. The first group was diagnosed as having developmental verbal dyspraxia. For the purpose of this paper, these are children with persisting speech difficulties in the absence of structural or obvious neurological damage. They may also be designated as having a phonological disorder. The second group of children had speech problems arising from structural abnormalities (cleft lip and palate). The children ranged in age from seven to eleven years and were administered tests of reading and spelling. The results indicated that children with developmental verbal dyspraxia were more at risk for specific reading and spelling problems than children with structural abnormality. When reading, the children with developmental verbal dyspraxia performed less well than age-matched controls and were unable to utilise a phonic strategy in order to tackle unfamiliar words. In fact they seemed to be guessing the targets from minimal visual features, for example 'canary' was read as 'competition', and 'think' as 'teacher'. When spelling, errors from the dyspraxic group were bizarre rather than logical, for example 'year' was spelt 'andere' and 'slippery' was 'greid'. In contrast, the children with structural abnormalities were not quantitatively or qualitatively different from age-matched normal controls. This suggests that it is a phonological disability rather than an articulatory difficulty that is the vulnerability factor when reading and spelling. In order to begin to understand why this might be so it is necessary to consider how a child learns to read and spell.

Normal and Abnormal Development of Reading and Spelling

Compare how the words CAT and YACHT might be read. If these words are familiar to the child they will have been stored in his orthographic lexicon and therefore could be accessed automatically. If, however, these are new words to the child he may try to apply grapheme–phoneme rules. This could be successful for CAT where there is one to one matching between letter and sound (c-a-t) but not for YACHT (y-a-ch-t) which would be pronounced as a rhyme of 'patched'. The child therefore needs at least two strategies to deal with reading words. The first is sound based and involves segmenting the word into its components and then blending the segments into the word as in a phonic approach to reading. The second is visually based and involves recognition of familiar words or patterns as in the look and say approach to reading. Without the first strategy children cannot tackle new or nonsense words and without the second strategy children cannot read familiar words automatically or irregular words.

Frith (1985) has presented a model to account for the development of these strategies in both reading and spelling. The model comprises three phases. The first, the *logographic* phase, occurs when a child recognises familiar words on the basis of minimal visual features. To move into the next phase, the *alphabetic,* a child must learn the relationship between letter and sounds. Once grapheme–phoneme rules are learned, new words can be tackled. Finally, in the *orthographic* phase a child's reading is independent of sound and there is automatic analysis of words into orthographic units, for example recognising that 'tion' at the end of 'addition' is pronounced 'shun'. This is therefore a morphemic rather than a phonemic phase. The same three phases are present in spelling development but the child does not necessarily pass through them at the same time when reading and spelling.

Frith suggests that 'classic' developmental dyslexia occurs when a child fails to break through to the alphabetic phase of literacy. Such an arrest would not preclude the child from progressing through the later phases of literacy development albeit more slowly or with obvious difficulties. If this alphabetic phase is such a stumbling block for dyslexic children with subtle speech problems, a pertinent question must be how do children with more obvious speech and language difficulties manage?

First, before embarking on reading and spelling specific words, the young child needs to develop an awareness of the purpose of written language. Reading readiness may be indicated by the child picking up a book or newspaper and 'reading' a familiar story or rhyme to an adult, pet or toy. Similarly, many adults have been the recipients of 'letters' from young children. These comprise a series of squiggles and shapes, often with a drawing, conveying the idea of communication (see Bissex, 1980). Children who have such metalinguistic awareness when starting school, have accelerated development of reading and spelling strategies (Francis, 1982). Children with delayed speech and language development may also be delayed in their metalinguistic development and therefore begin school at a disadvantage. In cases of environmental delay, however, there is no reason why the child should not catch up with his peers after appropriate or extra intervention and move through the phases of reading and spelling development smoothly, albeit more slowly.

As long as there are no visual perceptual deficits accompanying the speech and language handicap, even the most severe speech problem should not prevent a child from entering the logographic phase of reading and spelling, since this requires no sound skills. Normal children first recognise highly familiar words, such as store labels on bags, breakfast cereal or favourite chocolate bars. They are not able to read these words in different contexts or if written in a different script. This is essentially a whole word recognition phase. Reading skill is reliant on visual memory and visual errors are increasingly common.

The problem for the child with a specific speech disorder arises when he tries to break through to the alphabetic phase. This is when the relationship between letters and sounds is learned and unfamiliar words can be tackled via phoneme–grapheme translation rules. It is through the focused attention of learning letter names that children learn to discriminate and remember letter shapes. Furthermore, children associate the shape with a name that often incorporates the letter sound; for example, B/b, L/l, K/k. What is often viewed as a visual recognition task, learning letters, is an important grapheme–phoneme skill. The ability to make this association enables breakthrough into the alphabetic phase. Once children are able to utilise this phonological rather than visual strategy, they are in a position to invent spellings (see Read, 1975; Bissex, 1980). However, whereas alphabetic knowledge may be some guarantee for successful reading and spelling development in the normal child, this is not necessarily the case in the speech disordered population where there may be a problem abstracting the sounds and transferring the associated sounds/letters to the reading and spelling situation.

A Case of Arrested Reading and Spelling Development

Michael, aged 11 years, is a good example of a child stuck at the logographic stage. He was of normal intelligence but had a persisting speech problem of a dyspraxic nature. He had a reading age of 7;07 and a spelling age of 6;08. He had been educated in a language unit attached to a normal school since the age of six where he received regular speech therapy and remedial help. He could successfully identify letters by name and most by sound but could not use this knowledge to decipher or produce the written word. On a test of single word reading over 50% of his errors had a strong visual similarity to the target, for example, pint/paint, snail/nail, vase/varnish. The next highest proportion of errors (42%) were unsuccessful sound attempts where he tried to apply his phonics training but was unable to do so, for example, cask/atch, catch, ack, ask. Similarly, when spelling, errors were bizarre or nonphonetic indicating an inability to apply alphabetic skills, for example umbrella/rberherrelrarlsrllles, and cigarette/satesatarhaelerari.

Such nonphonetic spelling is characteristic of the logographic phase. On entering the alphabetic phase, spelling becomes semiphonetic and finally phonetic in nature (Ehri, 1985). Semiphonetic errors are partial word spellings usually found in pre- or beginner readers and include: a letter name to represent a sound (arm/RM), boundary sounds only (back/BK), vowels ignored or misrepresented unless their names can be used (boat/BOT), reduced clusters (crab/KB) and representation of syllables by graphemes (elephant/LFT). These errors show that the child can apply some alphabetic knowledge but does not have the tools or orthographic experience as yet, to represent what he has segmented. Phonetic spelling reflects increased orthographic experience. It is characterised by the one to one mapping of letters and sounds (cigarette/sigaret, catalogue/catalog). Sound blending is as important as sound segmentation. Without it, sound segmentation will not be helpful when decoding text as meanings cannot be accessed from a string of unrelated sounds.

In a recent study of spelling development in young school-age children, semiphonetic errors dominated the beginner spellers while phonetic errors were predominant in children with a spelling age of over eight years. Nonphonetic errors were minimal in these normally developing children. Michael's persisting visual errors when reading and his non-phonetic spelling is therefore a serious handicap indicating arrest in the logographic phase of reading and spelling.

What might explain this arrest in development? Two obvious possibilities will be explored: Input skills and Output skills. First, if a child is unable to discriminate between sounds then he is unlikely to remember them or associate the right sound with the letter shape. Michael, however could discriminate minimal pair words (pit/bit) on tests such as the Aston Index (Newton & Thomson, 1976), and the Wepman Auditory Discrimination Test (1958) but failed on tests comprising complex nonwords where detection of subtle sequencing changes was necessary, for example, ibikus/ikibus, wesp/weps. This has been followed up by Bridgeman & Snowling (1988) who tested twelve children in the age-range of seven to eleven years with developmental verbal dyspraxia, on an auditory discrimination task and compared their performance to reading age-matched controls. The task was designed to test sequential auditory discrimination in real and non words. Fifteen familiar and fifteen nonsense monosyllable word pairs, comprising cluster reversals (lots/lost, vost/vots) and the same number of word pairs without clusters (loss/lot, vos/vot) were randomly presented to the children. On the non-cluster word condition all the children were at ceiling. However, the dyspraxic children performed less well on the cluster reversal condition with a specific deficit on nonword items. Their performance cannot be explained by auditory perception alone since they were at ceiling on the non-cluster word condition. Neither can it be explained by orthographic experience since these children were matched on reading age. This supports the hypothesis that dyspraxic children are at risk on tasks of more complex auditory discrimination involving sequencing skill.

The second possibility is the child's output skills. To examine the relationship between children's speech and spelling performance, Snowling & Stackhouse (1983) examined a small group of dyspraxic children ranging in age from eight to ten years. Michael was included in this group. These children were matched on reading age with younger normally speaking children from the same school. Each child was asked to imitate, read, spell and copy a series of consonant–vowel–consonant syllables that varied in their degree of articulatory place change. For example, nil place change — mop, 1 place change — bat, 2 place changes — peg. Normal children were at ceiling on these tasks. The dyspraxic children performed within the same range as the controls on reading and copying but did significantly less well than the controls on imitation and spelling. A qualitative analysis of the imitation and spelling results was carried out to investigate the possible link between speech and spelling performance. Errors were categorised according to whether they differed from the correct form in voicing (dad/dat), placement (dog/dod) or manner (can/cal) of articulation. The findings were that accuracy of pronunciation did not guarantee correct spelling. Overall, there were more spelling than imitation errors but there was no obvious one to one relationship between the imitation and spelling errors.

During this study, it became apparent that the dyspraxic children had great difficulty in segmenting the target prior to spelling it. For example, 'Pam' was repeated correctly, segmented as 'pe-te' and spelled 'potm', 'Nick' was also repeated correctly, segmented as 'ke-ke-ne-i-te' and spelled 'cat'. This indicated a breakdown at the sound segmentation level prior to phoneme–grapheme translation. This observation is compatible with the results of the auditory discrimination tests. In order to identify whether complex nonwords are the same or different, the child needs to segment the words into their components in the right order.

If sound segmentation difficulties are at the root of the reading and spelling difficulties they should be demonstrated in more direct tests of segmentation. Michael is reported to have been delayed in his ability to segment words into syllables and received extra help with this. As a teenager he was still unable to play 'I Spy' and rhyming games successfully. When asked to produce rhyming words to targets, for example, cat/mat, he could only produce words that he had been taught in therapy. Less common words resulted in him producing either an alliteration (comb/come) or a semantic (wool/cotton) association with the target.

This segmentation difficulty also explains his spelling errors. For example, the bizarre spelling of 'cigarette' as 'satesatarhaelerari' is an unsuccessful attempt at sound segmentation. He transcribes each of his spelling attempts and backtracks several times. Dividing the word into three syllables $ci_1/gar_2/ette_3$, Michael's spelling can be explained as follows: $sa_1/te_3/s_1/at_3/ar_2/hael_2/er_2/ari_2$.

Unfortunately, because of the nature of Michael's speech problem, he cannot use articulation to help him segment words. The more he tries to repeat a word, the more variable it becomes. Furthermore, a lexical disorder is set up as words become wrongly accommodated in his orthographic lexicon. For example he was confident that 'organ' was 'orange' and is far more accepting of nonwords as real words than reading-age control children. In fact the concept of nonword was alien to him and indicated a persisting metalinguistic deficit.

Phonological Dyslexia

In summary, children with delayed speech and language development may begin school with a shaky foundation on which to map their written language skill. However, children with environmentally caused speech and language problems or children with articulatory difficulties arising from structural abnormalities should be no more at risk of specific reading and spelling difficulties than the non-speech and language handicapped population. Although they may progress more slowly they should pass through the normal order of reading and spelling phases outlined above. However, children with specific speech and language disorders of a phonological/dyspraxic nature are more at risk for a specific type of dyslexia, *phonological dyslexia,* characterised by an inability to break through or difficulty within the alphabetic phase of reading and spelling development. Central to this is an inability to segment and blend sounds. This difficulty first manifests itself when the child attempts to discriminate, sequence and programme articulation for speech and later when he attempts to read and spell. Michael is a good illustration of the range of difficulties experienced by such children but not all will be so severely impaired (see Snowling *et al.,* 1986).

Implications for the Professionals Involved

Finally, what are the implications of this research for the educational setting and the professionals involved? First, it suggests that one of the main aims of intervention with the young child is to enable him to develop and utilise alphabetic skills. A variety of auditory organisation and segmentation tasks can be used for this (see Stackhouse, 1985, for suggestions). Second, the acknowledgement of a relationship between spoken and written language calls into question the role of the speech therapist in reading and spelling disorders. The speech therapist clearly has a critical role in the child's preschool period of identifying the at risk child and promoting pre-reading and spelling skills since the dyslexics of the future are in speech therapy clinics now. Once the child goes to school speech therapists may carry out a liaison role with the teacher and advise on the individual child's needs. What is not so clear is the role of the speech therapist once the child's speech has improved to an acceptable level and yet the phonological deficit is still manifest in reading and spelling performance. Although I am reluctant to add more to the work of an already overloaded profession, caution is needed by therapists when discharging children with persisting phonological difficulties without ensuring adequate backup for their written language development. Close collaboration between speech therapists, teachers and psychologists is necessary if we are to understand and remediate the unfolding difficulties that speech disordered children experience in their spoken and written language development.

Acknowledgements

The author wishes to thank Bill Wells for his helpful comments on the paper and Maggie Snowling for her continuing support with this work.

References

BISSEX, G.L. 1980, *GNYS at Work: A Child Learns to Write and Read*. Cambridge, MA: Harvard University Press.

BRIDGEMAN, E. and SNOWLING, M. 1988, The perception of phoneme sequence: A comparison of dyspraxic and normal children. *British Journal of Disorders of Communication* 23, 3.

EHRI, L. 1985, Sources of difficulty in learning to spell and read. In M.L. WOLRAICH and D. ROUTH (eds). *Advances in Developmental and Behavioural Paediatrics*. Greenwich Conn.: Jai Press Inc.

FRANCIS, H. 1982, *Learning to Read*. London: George Allen and Unwin.

FRITH, U. 1985, Beneath the surface of developmental dyslexia. In K.E. PATTERSON, J.C. MARSHALL and M. COLTHEART (eds), *Surface Dyslexia*. London: Routledge and Kegan Paul.

INGRAM, T.T.S., MASON, A.W. and BLACKBURN, I. 1970, A retrospective study of 82 children with reading disability. *Developmental Medicine and Child Neurology* 12, 271–81.

MILES, T.R. 1982, *Dyslexia: The Pattern of Difficulties*. London: Granada.

NEWTON, M. and THOMSON, M.E. 1976, *The Aston Index*. Wisbech, Cambs: Learning Development Aids.

READ, C. 1975, Lessons to be learned from the preschool orthographer. In E.H. LENNEBERG and E. LENNEBERG (eds), *Foundations of Language Development* Vol. 2. London: Academic Press.

RUTTER, M. and YULE, W. 1973, Specific reading retardation. In L. MANN and D. SABATINO (eds), *The First Review of Special Education*. Philadelphia: Buttonwood Farms.

Snowling, M. and Stackhouse, J. 1983, Spelling performance of children with developmental verbal dyspraxia. *Developmental Medicine and Child Neurology* 25, 430–7.

Snowling, M., Stackhouse, J. and Rack, J. 1986, Phonological dyslexia and dysgraphia — a developmental analysis. *Cognitive Neuropsychology* 3(3), 309–40.

Stackhouse, J. 1982, An investigation of reading and spelling performance in speech disordered children. *British Journal of Disorders of Communication* 17(2), 53–60.

— 1985, Segmentation, speech and spelling difficulties. In M. Snowling (ed), *Children's Written Language Difficulties*. Windsor: NFER-Nelson.

Wepman, J.M. 1958, *Auditory Discrimination Test*. Chicago: University of Chicago Press.

3 The speech and language problems screening-test (SLPS)

JOANNE CORCORAN

The Speech and Language Problems Screening-Test (SLPS) has been developed by the Association for All Speech Impaired Children (AFASIC) and Leicester Polytechnic. SLPS is a school-age screening test designed to be used by teachers as an aid to identifying children with language impairments. The paper is divided into two sections. In the first section the need for a school-age language screening test will be outlined. In the second section considerations in the development of SLPS will be discussed, and the stages of test construction described.

Why Develop SLPS?

There is good reason to identify a language-impaired child given the well-documented relationship between language difficulties and later educational, emotional and social problems (Hall & Tomblin, 1978; Aram & Nation, 1980, 1984; King *et al.*, 1982; Baker & Cantwell, 1985). However, it is often extremely difficult to decide what constitutes a language problem. There are essentially two reasons for this difficulty; the first is the variation in normal language development. In general, research has concentrated on the variation in rate of language development. Studying the language development of pre-schoolers, Wells (1986) found that in a sample of 'normal' four-year-olds the difference between the most and least advanced children was 30–36 months. In addition to studies of rate of development, there has been interest in the variation in route of development. For example, Nelson (1978) found that children differed in the content of their early vocabulary. In this study one group of children had vocabularies mainly comprising words for objects, whereas another group used fewer object labels but more pronouns, modifiers and personal-social expressions. Such variability in both rate and route of language development makes it virtually impossible to draw a clear distinction between young children described as 'late developers' and children with significant language problems.

The second reason why identification may prove difficult relates to the fact that language impaired children are not a homogeneous group. The term 'language impaired' is a general label, and is used to refer to many types of impairments. A language impaired child may be one who has difficulty articulating sounds, or difficulty constructing the grammatical structures of the language. Equally, a language impaired child may be able to articulate sounds correctly, and be able to construct grammatical sentences, yet be unable to use language appropriately in a social context. As well as differences in the types of impairment, there are differences in the severity of language impairment. At one end of the scale there are children with severe problems. Depending on the definition of moderate to severe language impairment employed, estimates of prevalence vary from approximately 1 to 4% (Ingram, 1963; Rutter *et al.*, 1970; Morley, 1972; Fundudis *et al.*, 1979; Silva *et al.*, 1983; Richman *et al.*, 1982; Drillen & Drummond, 1983). The nature of these severe to moderate problems means that they are obvious and as such it is highly likely that they will be identified at an early age. At the other end of the scale there are children with less severe, more subtle problems. These problems are less likely to be identified in the pre-school period. In school a child with a language problem may appear shy or withdrawn, have difficulty making friends, or be described as a 'loner'. Alternatively a child may behave in a hostile and aggressive manner. Although these secondary problems may be obvious, the underlying language problem may be missed. Of studies examining the prevalence of any language impairment, Chazan (1983) reported that 11% of school-age children were experiencing some form of language difficulty. The National Child Development Study (Davie *et al.*, 1972; Peckham, 1973) produced comparable results; in this study school medical officers assessed 14% of seven-year-old children as having speech and language problems, teachers reported 11% of children 'difficult to understand because of poor speech'. Crystal (1984) suggests that 10% of school-age children have a language handicap which is sufficiently serious to pose them and their caretakers problems. If this is the case, mainstream teachers can expect to have 2–3 children in their class who are experiencing some form of language impairment.

Given the inherent difficulties in identifying children with language impairments, how well prepared are teachers to recognise these children?

To be well prepared in the task of recognising language problems a teacher has to be aware of the stages of normal language development, the role of individual differences in language and the range of language difficulties. Unfortunately there is some evidence that teacher-training courses may not adequately prepare teachers for identifying and working with a language impaired child. The Warnock Report (DES, 1978), considering the needs of children with language difficulties, commented that 'the special needs of this group are slowly becoming recognized and understood . . . there has been a growth in the provision in recent years but no corresponding development in teacher-training'. The report went on to recommend that teacher-training courses should include more input on the identification and education of children with special needs in the mainstream school. In recent study by Lesser and Hassip (1986), a number of professional groups, who were all potential referrers to speech therapy services, were questioned about their knowledge of speech therapy. The study revealed that many teachers had received very little formal teaching on speech and language impairments during their training courses. It was also found that of the professional groups, which included health visitors and doctors, teachers were the least well informed about the work of speech therapists and generally unaware of the potential help available from speech therapists on language, reading and spelling problems. There has to be some doubt as to how representative these findings are, as the study included only a small sample of subjects per professional group. If representative, the findings suggest that the recommendations of the Warnock Report have not been implemented and some courses remain deficient in input on language development and disorders.

It is apparent that there is a need for a school-age language screening test. Many children experiencing language problems, particularly those with severe problems, are indeed identified in the pre-school period. Unfortunately many other children enter school with undetected language problems. When this occurs the task of recognition and identification falls largely on the classroom teacher. This task is by no means straightforward, and there is some evidence that teacher-training courses leave teachers singularly unprepared for such a task.

The Development and Construction of SLPS

When developing a test it is important to be clear about the purpose that the test will serve. All psychometric tests are tools that can 'inform, but not supplant, the professional judgments of teachers' (Sumner, 1987). SLPS is a screening test and as such it is not designed to be used as a diagnostic instrument, nor a definitive guide to a child's language functioning. Screening tests are used for two distinct purposes; for predicting and for confirming problems. In education, predictive screening involves the employment of psychometric tests to identify children who are likely to fail at school. The theory is that once a child has been identified as being 'at risk', appropriate intervention can be implemented in order to prevent future difficulties. Alternatively screening tests are used to assess a child's current functioning and to confirm any existing problems. In common with pre-school language screening tests, SLPS is intended to be used to confirm that a child has language difficulties. It is designed for use by teachers as an aid to structuring observations, focusing upon aspects of a child's language development and making decisions as to the need for referral to a speech therapist for more detailed assessment.

In the development of a test, the criteria by which the test will be ultimately evaluated have to be considered throughout. To be useful, a screening test has to be effective. Effectiveness refers to the accuracy and validity of the test. Law (1987) suggests that the problem of the validity of a screening test can be reduced to two questions;

(1) Is the test specific? i.e. are the children who are picked out by the test identified correctly?
(2) Is the test sensitive? i.e. are the children not picked out by the test free from language impairment?

The levels of test specificity and sensitivity are related to the setting of the cut-off point on the test, above which it is recommended that a child be referred for further assessment. If a test has a low cut-off point, there is a risk that the test will be insufficiently specific, and children with no language problems will be wrongly identified by the test. Misidentification of this nature could result in a number of adverse consequences including unnecessary anxiety on the part of the child and his parents, ill-founded expectations of the child on the part of teachers, and wasted time and resources on the part of all the professionals involved. On the other hand, if a test has a high cut-off point, there is the possibility that the test will be insufficiently sensitive and that children with significant language problems will be missed by the test. Again, potentially harmful effects could be the result. As noted earlier, a child who proceeds through school with an undetected language problem is at risk of experiencing further educational and social difficulties. When deciding where to set the cut-off point on the test there are no fixed rules, and the final decision has to be made by weighing up the risks and costs of misidentification versus non-identification.

As well as being effective, a screening test has to be efficient. Efficiency refers to how easy and straightforward a test is to use. If a test is inefficient it will not be used because it is too difficult to understand, or too time-consuming to complete. Obviously to some extent the two criteria of effectiveness and efficiency are at odds: an effective test is likely to be a reasonably long and detailed test, in contrast an efficient test is likely to be a simple and quick instrument. It is important that neither effectiveness nor efficiency are sacrificed in the development of a screening test. A test may be accurate but is the test suitable for use in the classroom? Similarly, although a 'slick and quick' test is easy to use, does it reliably identify children with language problems? Throughout the construction of SLPS this problem has been recognised and attempts made to maximise both effectiveness and efficiency.

Turning to the stages of test construction, there have been essentially three stages in the development of SLPS. Work on SLPS was first initiated by the charity Association For All Speech Impaired Children (AFASIC). The aim of the work was to devise a language screening test to be used with children aged five to eleven years. A panel of professional workers worked on the construction of such a test, and produced a 94 item questionnaire. For each of the 94 items on the questionnaire, the teacher had to decide whether the item generally applied to the child, sometimes applied to the child, or never applied to the child. The questionnaire was organised into eight subsections: Response to Sound, Movement and Motor Skill, Social Communication, Play and Recreation, Learning Behaviour, Errors in Sound, Vocabulary and Grammar. Language does not develop in isolation and it would be artificial to consider it separate from other aspects of a child's development, hence the sections on motor skills, social functioning and cognitive abilities as well as sections obviously related to speech and language. Once the questionnaire had been constructed, AFASIC proceeded to organise a validation study on the test. This study involved using the questionnaire with an experimental group of children (i.e. children with known language problems) and a control group of children (i.e. children with no known language problems). Using this methodology it would be possible to assess how well the questionnaire discriminated between these two groups of children. It is a truism to say that validation is a crucial stage in the development of every psychometric test. Despite this it is not uncommon for a test to be poorly evaluated or not evaluated at all. A large number of pre-school language screening tests are developed by individual health authorities for their own purposes. Due to constraints on personnel, time and money these tests are rarely evaluated. Yet without evaluation it is impossible to assess the effectiveness of the test in terms of specificity and sensitivity.

During the second stage of development Leicester Polytechnic became involved with the construction of SLPS. During this stage the data from the AFASIC validation study was analysed. The results indicated that the questionnaire consistently and accurately distinguished between the experimental and control groups (Hiles & Rowley, 1985). Such findings suggested that the AFASIC screen was a valid instrument for identifying children with speech and language problems. Although the test was found to be effective, a 94 item test could hardly be described as efficient. To improve efficiency the test was revised into a shorter version, referred to as the pilot version of SLPS. This process of revision primarily involved the statistical technique of item analysis to isolate and then eliminate the test items that were not contributing to the discriminatory power of the test. As the only items omitted were those that weakly discriminated between the experimental and control groups, this process of shortening the test did not detract from the effectiveness of the test (Hiles & Rowley, 1985). The final result of the revision was a 56 item checklist, that remained organised in the original eight sub-sections. To illustrate the format and content of this pilot version of SLPS, one sub-section of the test is reprinted in Figure 1. It was in this format that AFASIC published the pilot test, Speech and Language Problems Screening-Test.

In the third stage of development the efficiency of the pilot version of SLPS was considered. To do this, teachers, speech therapists and

MOVEMENT AND MOTOR SKILLS

		G.A.	*S.A.*	*N.A.*
1.	*Seems unaware of a runny nose.*	[ ]	[ ]	[ ]
2.	*Has poor co-ordination, e.g. delayed in using alternate feet downstairs, delayed in hopping on one foot, or delayed in kicking a ball.*	[ ]	[ ]	[ ]
3.	*Is clumsy, e.g. bumps into things, falls down often.*	[ ]	[ ]	[ ]
4.	*Finds judging speed and distance difficult, e.g. catching.*	[ ]	[ ]	[ ]
5.	*Developmentally delayed in establishing dominance, i.e. laterality and handedness.*	[ ]	[ ]	[ ]
6.	*Poor pencil control.*	[ ]	[ ]	[ ]
7.	*Poor eye-hand co-ordination, e.g. finds use of scissors difficult.*	[ ]	[ ]	[ ]
			Total for this section	[ ]

FIGURE 1 *Movement and Motor Skills sub-section of the pilot version*

educational psychologists who had used the pilot SLPS were approached and asked for their comments on the test. Despite the enthusiasm many professionals expressed for such a school-age screening test, the feedback indicated that there were problems with the pilot test. A major problem was the age range of the test, 5.0–11.0 years. Obviously there are vast differences between the behaviour of a five-year-old and an eleven-year-old, so it was hardly surprising that some of the items were considered to be inappropriate for certain age groups. Other criticisms centred on the length of the test (56 items were still considered to be too many), the rather complicated scoring system and the fact that the wording of a number of items was vague and overly technical. Finally the presentation and printing of the pilot SLPS is rather poor. Although this problem can be easily remedied, it is worth stressing the importance of presentation. Unless a screen is attractive to the user, in the sense that it immediately looks simple and straightforward, it is unlikely to promote confidence on the part of the user.

To overcome the difficulties with the pilot version of the test, the original validation study data were reanalysed. On the basis of this further analysis a second version was produced, referred to as the experimental version of SLPS. An important change with the experimental version of SLPS is that the age range is narrower; it is for use with children aged 6.0–10.0 years. Other changes include the simplification of the scoring system from the original three-category system ('does the item generally, sometimes or never apply to the child') to a two-category system whereby the

MOVEMENT AND MOTOR SKILLS

1. Finds judging speed and distance difficult, e.g. catching. ☐
2. Developmentally delayed in establishing preference for either the right or left hand/foot etc. ☐
3. Delayed in developing self-help skills, e.g. has problems with dressing, eating, washing. ☐
4. Has poor pencil control. ☐
5. Has poor co-ordination, e.g. delayed in using alternate feet downstairs, delayed in hopping on one foot or kicking a ball. ☐

TOTAL FOR THIS SECTION ☐

FIGURE 2 *Movement and Motor Skills sub-section of the experimental version of SLPS.*

scorer has to decide whether or not the item applies to the child. Also there are fewer items, the wording has been clarified and the general presentation made clearer and more straightforward. The complete experimental version is 40 items long, five items per each of the eight sections. To provide a comparison between the pilot and experimental versions of the test, the Movement and Motor Skills sub-section of the experimental version of the test is reprinted in Figure 2. It is hoped that this version of SLPS will be an easier and quicker test to use. At present this experimental version of SLPS is being evaluated in a national study. The results of the study will be used to assess if indeed the test is efficient, while continuing to be an accurate indicator of language problems.

A copy of the pilot version of SLPS can be obtained from AFASIC.

References

ARAM, D.M. and NATION, J.E. 1980, Preschool language disorders and subsequent language and academic difficulties. *Journal of Communication Disorders* 13, 159–70.

ARAM, D.M., EKELMAN, B.L. and NATION, J.E. 1984, Preschoolers with language disorders: Ten years later. *Journal of Speech and Hearing Research* 27, 234–44.

BAKER, L. and CANTWELL, D.P. 1985, Psychiatric and learning disorders in children with speech and language disorders: A critical review. *Advances in Learning and Behavioural Disabilities* 4, 1–28.

CHAZAN, M. 1983, *Some of Our Children, the Education of Children with Special Needs.* London: Open Books.

CRYSTAL, D. 1984, *Language Handicap in Children.* Stratford-upon-Avon: National Council for Special Education.

DAVIE, R., BUTLER, N. and GOLDSTEIN, H. 1972, *From Birth to Seven.* London: Longman.

DES 1978, *Special Educational Needs: Report of the Committee of Enquiry into the Education of Handicapped Children and Young Persons.* Warnock Report. London: HMSO.

DRILLEN, C. and DRUMMOND, M. 1983, *Development Screening and the Child with Special Needs.* Clinics in Developmental Medicine No. 86. London: Heinemann Medical Books.

FUNDUDIS, T., KOLVIN, I. and GARSIDE, R. (eds) 1979, *Speech Retarded and Deaf Children: their Psychological Development.* London: Academic Press.

HALL, P.K. and TOMBLIN, J.B. 1978, A follow-up study of children with articulation and language disorders. *Journal of Speech and Hearing Disorders* 43, 227–41.

HILES, D.R. and ROWLEY, D.T. 1985, *Validity study of AFASIC's 'Speech and Language Problems Screening test (SLPS)'.* Unpublished report, Leicester Polytechnic.

INGRAM, T.T.S. 1963, Report of the dysphasia sub-committee of the Scottish Paediatric Society, Unpublished. Reported in A. WEBSTER and C. MCCONNELL 1987, *Special Needs in Ordinary Schools: Children With Speech and Language Difficulties.* London: Cassell Educational Ltd.

KING, R.R., JONES, C. and LASKY, E. 1982, In retrospect, a 15-year follow-up of speech-language disordered children. *Language, Speech and Hearing Services in Schools* 13, 24–32.

Law, J. 1987, Early language screening: Towards a methodology. *College of Speech Therapists Bulletin* No. 421, 1–2.

Lesser, R. and Hassip, S. 1986, Knowledge and opinions of speech therapy in teachers, doctors and nurses. *Child: Care, Health and Development* 12, 235–49.

Morley, M. 1972, *The Development and Disorders of Speech in Childhood,* 3rd edn. Edinburgh: Churchill Livingstone.

Nelson, K. 1978, Individual differences in language development: Implications for development and language. *Developmental Psychology* 17(2), 170–87.

Peckham, C.S. 1973, Speech defects in a national sample of children aged seven years. *British Journal of Disorders of Communication* 8(2), 2–7.

Richman, N., Stevenson, J.E. and Graham, P.J. 1982, *Pre-school to School: A Behavioural Study.* London: Academic Press.

Rutter, M., Tizard, J. and Whitmore, K. 1970, *Education, Health and Behaviour.* London: Longman.

Silva, P.A., McGee, R. and Williams, S.M. 1983, Developmental language delay from 3 to 7 years and its significance for low intelligence and reading difficulties at age 7. *Developmental Medicine and Child Neurology* 25, 783–93.

Sumner, R. 1987, *The Role of Testing in Schools.* London: NFER-Nelson.

Wells, G. 1986, Variation in child language. In P. Fletcher and M. Garman (eds), *Language Acquisition,* 2nd edn. Cambridge: Cambridge University Press.

4 Screening and intervention with children with speech and language difficulties in mainstream schools

ANN LOCKE

There appears to be a growing awareness within the state education system of children who have difficulty acquiring or using spoken language. Figures for the incidence of these problems are still scarce, coming from a relatively small number of surveys carried out over the past 40 years. Such studies have produced widely varying figures ranging from less than 1 in 1000 to more than 20 in 100 children having difficulty with communication at some time in their school life. A useful review of these surveys can be found in Webster and McConnell's book *Special Needs in Ordinary Schools — Children with Speech and Language Difficulties* (1987). The general picture that emerges suggests that around 1 child in every 1000 is likely to have severe difficulty in acquiring spoken language; 1 child in 100 will have difficulty that seriously affects his/her education; and some 10 children in 100 may have difficulties that could interfere with their educational progress at some time.

Projecting these figures onto the primary school population of England, Scotland and Wales, currently around four million children, suggests that some 4000 children are likely to have difficulties of such severity that they will need some period of full time special educational help if they are to have a chance of making reasonable progress in school. The most recent figures of children receiving such help show that in 1985 some 2500 children were being educated in specialist schools or units (Hutt & Donlan, 1987). Though the number of such specialist educational places still seems to be increasing there are, nevertheless, likely to be some 1000 or more children with severe problems currently being educated in mainstream schools. In addition there are likely to be some 40,000 children in the mainstream system whose problems are less severe but still serious enough to interfere with their educational progress, presenting a major problem to their class teachers.

Birmingham, with a current school population of around 100,000 primary age children, could expect to identify around 100 children with severe difficulties. Eighty children are at present being educated in the six nursery and primary language units being run by the local education authority. In addition some 1000 children, potentially 2 or 3 in each of the city's 450 nursery classes and primary schools, are likely to be experiencing particular difficulty establishing educational skills as a result of their speech and/or language impairment.

In 1985 Birmingham Education Authority implemented plans to address this problem by appointing a teacher to one of its support services, the Visiting Teacher Service, to set up a system for helping children with speech and language impairments in mainstream schools. It was clear from the start that such a system would have to be school-based, to meet the needs of the potentially significant numbers of children involved, and to be compatible with the general move towards helping the majority of children with special needs within mainstream schools.

Three major issues need to be addressed in setting up such a system: how to identify the children in question; how to intervene effectively; how to evaluate the procedures. All three issues present immediate practical problems. The initial aim of the procedure is the early identification of children with serious speech or language difficulties. Quite large numbers of young children however have poor communication skills, especially when they first start school. But only a small proportion of these children are likely to need help for more than a year or two. Predicting longer term problems from the initial group presenting difficulties is both time consuming and, perhaps more importantly, unreliable. An initial screen, therefore, should not attempt to do this but simply be a means of bringing to the class teacher's attention any child who is not communicating as often or as effectively as the majority of children in the class. With all the children in the class to be considered, the screening procedure should not require extensive explanation. It should be relatively quick and easy to implement, and make use of the teacher's everyday observations of the child's language skills.

The identification of any learning difficulty is of limited value if the teacher is not given some fairly prompt help to deal with the problem in the classroom. Significant numbers of children may be identified by the type of wide screening procedure suggested, and all these children should receive some kind of help whether their difficulties are later shown to be serious or not. A few may receive speech therapy; all still spend most of their time with the class teacher so it is in the classroom that intervention should be made available, and the class teacher will have the responsibility for providing it. The only way this can be done is by making use of skills teachers already have, highlighting those aspects of good classroom practice which benefit all children's communication skills and discussing how a small additional input may be sufficient to enable many children to settle down and communicate effectively.

The ultimate aim of a screening and intervention programme is the early identification of children with difficulties. If oral language problems are not recognised early in school life, children may not be seen as having special needs until they show behavioural difficulties or fail to read in later years. Only time will tell whether such an early identification procedure will reduce the number of children with behavioural or reading problems stemming from poor oral language skills. More immediately, the procedure should provide a quick and effective way of reassessing the children first identified, to indicate those who need no further help and those who appear to have more serious problems.

These are the considerations that have shaped the development of the Birmingham Primary Intervention Procedures, for children with speech and language impairments. Good classroom practice underlies all aspects of these procedures and is based on the following six principles.

First is the skill of the teacher in promoting a positive relationship with all the children in her class, so that each child is happy and therefore receptive to learning.

Second is the need to provide an active learning environment, so that children are not expected to spend all day sitting at a table but are given regular opportunities to move about and learn through 'doing'.

Third, the learning of all children will be enhanced if the teacher promotes a theme-based, integrated curriculum so that ideas and information introduced in one curriculum area, e.g. Maths, are illustrated and expanded in others, such as P.E. and Art and Craft.

Fourth, children's use of oral language should be encouraged as a priority. Children promote their own learning through language, talking to themselves and others as they meet new experiences. Talking should be seen as a fundamental way in which children clarify their ideas and solve problems.

Fifth, the education provided in any school will be improved if the staff follows an agreed set of written objectives. The writing of such objectives should promote a comprehensive review of teaching methods within the school and provide a framework for consistent teaching.

Such objectives will also enable the sixth principle of good teaching practice to be implemented, the keeping of school-based records.

It requires considerable time and good organisation to implement and follow these principles but once established, a school will be well able to meet the problems presented by children with special educational needs.

Birmingham Primary Intervention Procedures for Children with Speech and Language Impairment.

The following account outlines the system as it is currently being implemented in ten primary schools. The schools were all invited to be involved following input from members of the Visiting Teacher Service in connection with individual children. Some schools implement the system throughout their infant department; some involve reception classes only; others have left the choice to individual teachers. All schools are asked to support the system for at least a year in the first instance. During that time a teacher from the Visiting Teacher Service visits the school at four to six weekly intervals to discuss the progress of the children with their teachers.

The numbering of stages of the procedure has recently been modified following discussion with educational psychologists currently running in service courses on special needs for all Birmingham mainstream schools. The content and progression of stages still follows the outline given in Newcastle on 23 April 1988.

Stage 1. First level procedures

1a. Initial Identification

The initial identification involves a 4–6 week period of school based observation. Teachers are asked to fill in, on a grid provided, the names of all children showing any of the behaviours on the screening checklist. See Figure 1. Degree of difficulty is not specified; if a child's behaviour is a cause of concern to the teacher, then s/he should be included.

Ideally this screen takes place in September, and all children causing concern should be identified by the first half term.

FIGURE 1 *Visiting teacher service — Primary schools project, speech and language*

Primary Screening Procudure

I. *IDENTIFICATION*

Behavioural indicators of possible adjustment, oral language, sensory (hearing and vision), motor, and learning difficulties.

Please list all children who show any of the following behaviours.

1. Is socially isolated
2. Says little to anyone
3. Shows aggressive/spiteful behaviour towards others
4. Is difficult to understand
5. Rarely uses sentences of more than a few words
6. Uses sentences that are grammatically incorrect; language sounds 'babyish'
7. Is particularly reluctant to ask and/or answer questions with an adult

8. Responds inconsistently to spoken instructions
9. Regularly appears to 'switch-off' or lose concentration in an oral teaching context
10. Regularly but inconsistently, gives inappropriate response to verbal comment, instructions or questioning
11. Shows more than average anxiety or embarrassment if singled out from a group
12. Seeks constant reassurance from teacher and/or other children that his/her behaviour is acceptable

13. Does not always do as s/he is told, but is inconsistent in response
14. Whole body movements are clumsy/poorly co-ordinated
15. Has poor hand control e.g. in drawing and writing
16. Please add any other behaviours that give cause for concern

---

1b. Initial intervention

Initial intervention involves two broad approaches with all children identified: managing the child in the classroom and the promotion of those low-key educational approaches that are likely to benefit all the children involved. Teachers are asked to implement these strategies for a minimum of 2–3 months.

Aspects of good management can be summarised under three areas

(a) *Building the child's self-confidence*

Strategies should include giving each child a small amount of individual attention every day; fostering his/her relationships with other children; encouraging each child to take some special responsibility; and highlighting skills the child does well.

(b) *Dealing with the effects of particular problems in the classroom*

Handouts are provided for teachers, outlining various ways in which particular difficulties, for example, unclear speech, can be minimised in the classroom.

(c) *Obtaining background information*

Sources of background information include parents, previous school records, medical records, or direct contact with other agencies e.g. speech therapy service. Relevant information may include evidence of a previous conductive hearing loss, previous speech therapy intervention etc. Contact with parents, where appropriate, can be particularly useful.

Low key educational approaches

The educational approaches suggested at the first level of intervention are based on the six principles of good teaching practice outlined above together with a small number of specific teaching strategies.

Specific teaching strategies

Five specific teaching strategies are discussed with teachers. They are not expected to use all approaches with all children but to try those they feel would be most compatible with their own teaching style and best meet the needs of particular children. The most important consideration is that all children receive some individual attention every day.

1. *Increasing incidental conversation*

Teachers are encouraged to look for ways in which they can increase children's involvement in incidental conversation. Strategies are discussed with all adults who provide any input to the class and children are grouped wherever possible with other children who will talk with them but not dominate the conversation.

2. *Providing opportunities for listening activities*

Ways in which children are expected to listen such as, attending to stories, learning rhymes by heart, establishing early phonic skills, are discussed with teachers. All children identified will benefit from regular opportunities to be involved in these and other listening activities, particularly in small group sessions. In these sessions they can either repeat activities carried out with the class as a whole, or have early exposure to new activities.

3. *Promoting the learning of new vocabulary*

A range of vocabulary, particularly verbs, adjectives and prepositions should be identified, highlighted and used repeatedly in ongoing cross-curricular theme work. Displaying a written list of such vocabulary enables all adults and older children involved with the class to use these words regularly in their conversations with the identified group.

4. *Promoting oral language use across all areas of the curriculum*

All areas of the curriculum can be used to promote conversation e.g. reasoning skills can be promoted in Maths — comparing and classifying objects, and in Science — understanding cause and effect. The ability to report previous experience can be developed during art and craft, science, after outings, cookery. The use of imaginative language can be promoted in imaginative play sessions, role play activities, story telling.

5. *Promoting self-organisation and pre-literacy skills*

The use of individual activity boxes is suggested for children who are making slow progress in literacy skills. A small selection of pre-reading or writing activities in these boxes are given to children while others in the class are involved in more formal literacy activities. Children are initially expected to complete these tasks on their own. With practice they can be encouraged to fill their own activity box and keep themselves busy while the teacher is occupied.

If some of the general procedures and specific teaching strategies outlined above are implemented consistently for 2–3 months most of the children initially identified should have settled into the class and have started to make educational progress.

At a time that is convenient for the teacher, at the beginning of the Spring term or perhaps before the second half-term holiday, the third part of the first level procedure should be carried out.

1c. First level evaluation

After a reasonable period of intervention the teacher should reassess all the children identified on the original checklist, first using a new grid, then comparing the results with the original observations.

The following patterns of behaviour are likely to be indicated:

(1) Children who have improved so much that no further special attention is considered necessary.
(2) Children who are making progress but who still require first level interventions.
(3) Children who need attention in other areas, for example eye–hand co-ordination skills, with or without additional help with oral language.
(4) Children added to the system, either because they are new to a class, or because the teacher now considers they would benefit from additional help.
(5) Children who are making little progress and are still causing concern.

Stage 2. Second level procedures

The procedure outlined in 1c. above, First Level Evaluation, also provides the procedure for identifying children who should be considered for the more focused language work of Level 2, i.e. those children who have made little or no progress. The numbers of such children in any class or even school should be small. So although the procedures outlined at Level 2 are time consuming to implement it is hoped they will not place too much demand on the resources a school can provide for children with special needs.

2b. Second level intervention

Profiling and focused language work

The aim of intervention in classroom and small group work should be to promote the balanced development of the child. Teaching those skills the child finds difficult should be guided by the following principles:

(1) Most of the time children with learning difficulties do not need different teaching techniques but a great deal more of the same approach that helps all children to learn. More input and time is needed to help the children acquire skills and to learn to use them in a wide variety of settings, before moving on to the teaching of more complex skills.

(2) Small group work, where the practice of overlearning suggested above can go on, is, therefore, an essential element in the learning opportunities offered to these children.

(3) Children often fail to learn because information is presented to them in too complex a form; ideas are explained through talk alone or simply with reference to pictures, with no opportunity for children to become involved in concrete situations with real objects. The more difficulty a child is having learning any skill, the more the learning environment should encourage him to be physically involved i.e. to use his whole body to promote learning. For example, children do not initially learn spatial concepts by moving objects around a table or by just looking at pictures; they learn them by moving themselves around objects and people. Stages of conceptual learning are outlined in Figure 2.

(4) As children progress through school, the majority are increasingly able to move through the stages of conceptual learning outlined in Figure 2 and gradually miss some out altogether. Children with learning difficulties cannot 'short-cut' this progression and may need to follow it carefully in every area of new learning. They regularly need new skills to be broken down into small steps before they are able to make progress.

FIGURE 2 *Stages of concept learning*

1. Whole body + talk
2. Eyes and hands — 3 D + talk
3. Eyes and hands — 2 D + talk
4. Eyes only — pictures + talk
5. Eyes only — schematic + talk
6. Talk only

Intervention at Level 2 includes four steps: finding out more about the child's overall development; planning an intervention programme based on a detailed assessment of language and other educational skills; setting up a timetable for small group teaching; and evaluating the child's ongoing learning.

Programmes of this type will need to be implemented for at least 3–6 months or the rest of the academic year. For some children, this approach may prove to be the only way they are able to make progress in the mainstream setting.

(a) *Finding out more about a child's overall development*

A range of teaching materials have been developed by the Birmingham Visiting Teacher Service which enable the class teacher to make a detailed assessment of a child's overall development. The teacher can profile maturational and educational development in some detail in order to identify particular skills that need to be promoted. These include listening and comprehension skills as well as language use skills.

(b) *Planning intervention*

Intervention for children should address the following issues: those management strategies that help the child to function confidently in the class should be continued; ongoing teaching should aim to promote the balanced development of an individual child. The materials used in (a) above to assess the child's maturational and educational development will help identify a child's strengths and weaknesses, and thus can form the basis of an individual teaching programme. Detailed work on specific aspects of comprehension and language use should be planned for small group sessions led by an adult. Objectives set for these sessions should be repeated and consolidated in general classroom activities.

(c) *Timetabling for small group work*

The timetabling of sessions for small group work should be organised for the school as a whole if possible to make the best use of people, places and time. A minimum of two small group sessions a week will be needed to promote learning, particularly language learning, in children requiring Level 2 intervention.

(d) *Evaluation of ongoing learning*

Careful checking of the child's learning of new skills, especially in areas of marked difficulty, should be a routine part of the teaching strategies used at Stage 2. Regular rechecking of skills learnt should be carried out at the beginning of each new term and skills not established should be practised again. The maturational and educational profiles can be used for this purpose.

The procedures outlined in the second level of intervention should be continued for the rest of the school year. Only then can any realistic evaluation be made of the school's ability to meet the child's special educational needs.

2c. Second level evaluation

Stage 2 evaluation should be carried out with all children involved in the second level intervention procedures, some three months after these have been implemented, and before the end of that school year. The aim of this evaluation is to check the following criteria:

(1) That the child comes willingly to school, is reasonably well integrated and relates acceptably with his peers.

(2) The child is making some progress in all areas of the curriculum.

(3) The child's position in the class is not significantly below the slowest learning group of children.

This information should be assembled by all those teachers who have regular contact with the child, using school records, the profiles provided with these procedures, the original checklist of identifying behaviours as well as the verbal impressions of those adults who know the child well, including his parents.

If a child meets all these criteria, the school has done well to meet his/her needs, and hopefully will be able to maintain the child for at least another year. If any one is not being met, some discussion should be set up to consider what changes could be implemented to improve the situation. If only one, or none of these criteria are met, the school should seriously consider whether they are able to meet the needs of that child for another year, or whether they should ask for a psychological assessment, with a view to asking for the child to be statemented.

Stage 3. Referral For Psychological Assessment

Referral for psychological assessment should be considered for any child not meeting the continuation criteria outlined after a period of Level 2 intervention. At least six months intervention should be implemented before this is considered; but realistically a year's focused language intervention may be necessary before a child shows significant improvement. Occasionally a child may show such complex problems that the school will feel the need for psychological assessment long before a year has passed. The headteacher should be able to call for this as soon as it is thought to be necessary.

Procedures involved in this process, and the additional help that will be offered following such assessment differ widely across the country.

Conclusion

The Birmingham Primary Intervention Procedures have now been in operation for three years. Four schools have been involved from the start; one dropped out with pressure of existing work, the other three are still using the procedures. Seven more schools have joined the pilot project and all ten schools have indicated their interest in continuing the procedures next year. Several more schools have expressed a wish to initiate this work in September.

During the last academic year the Visiting Teacher Service had the opportunity of running, as part of G.R.I.S.T., a six-week course to support the project. This was found to be most productive for teachers and, ideally, provision should be made in future to include course work as a regular part of the procedures.

While the teachers involved consider the framework for these procedures to be reasonably well established, there is still a need for the development of materials to support classroom practice, particularly with those children having serious difficulties. All that is needed now is the time to complete this work and the means of making it available to other interested teachers!

References

Hutt, E. and Donlan, C. 1987, *A Survey of Language Units.* London: ICAN.

Webster, A. and McConnell, C. 1987, *Special Needs in Ordinary Schools: Children with Speech and Language Difficulties.* London: Cassell Educational.

5 Staged assessment in literacy: implications for language problems in secondary schools

MICHAEL BEVERIDGE

Literacy in Primary and Secondary Schools: The Educational Context

Many young children who have problems with spoken language will, when they reach school age, also have difficulty with reading and writing (Lee & Shapiro-Fine, 1984). Unfortunately, when their reading and writing problems emerge, many of these children will not be identified as having an underlying language disability. This is partly because, in many cases, their difficulties in school will not be restricted to literacy. Because language and communication are so crucial for educational progress these children will usually find difficulty with most aspects of school learning. And because their basic problem has not been recognised as linguistic they are often misleadingly labelled as 'slow learners'.

In many cases spoken language difficulties are effectively resolved during the primary school years. But because of the increasing emphasis on the written word, literacy problems remain. This paper looks, in particular, at the continuing problems that these children have with literacy in secondary school and shows how the recent Staged Assessments in Literacy Project (SAIL) is able to identify and suggest additional ways of helping these children.

The piece of writing shown in Figure 1 was produced by a child taking part in the initial SAIL assessments, prior to which his school had no record of, or plans to alleviate his difficulties. Figure 1 was collected during the trial phase of the SAIL scheme in which more than 2,000 children were assessed. This sample produced many examples of children's writing which were clearly indicative of a level of skill below that needed to succeed in the secondary school system. Many of the children in the pilot assessment were in clear need of remedial help but were lost in the education system without support for their language difficulties.

Last monday I was sorting
socks out A man went to the
other assistant please tal me
were the shoes are the assistant
said go and find they. The man
said I went wanted to see
the manager. The shop assitant
he is not in the man said
I walk want the assistant said
you weth had a long want so
get lost the man said not sad
that the assisttant get go off
there shop I went to see the
manager no I said he is not
in well I auth want the manager
walked in the shop. I said the
shop assistant told me to get
lost I want to no were the
shoes was the manager said
sead say sorry the shop assistant
said sorry. I well take you to
the shoes.

FIGURE 1. *Example of writing produced by a child with no previously identified literacy problem.*

Later in this paper I will outline part of the SAIL scheme and its potential for use in understanding the problems of language disabled children. First, however, there are some important issues about the way responsibility for literacy needs to be reorganised in the secondary education system. Without major changes in the assignment of responsibilities, language problems will continue to be unidentified and children will fail to cope with the literacy demands of secondary schools.

Why are children whose writing, and also reading, is in need of remedial assistance currently often not being identified and helped? There are several reasons, the most important of which are (1) the absence of a coherent cross-curricular policy on literacy and (2) a general lack of awareness of language structure and function in relation to secondary school learning. Before discussing the SAIL scheme in relation to the second of these points, a brief analysis of the current situation with regard to secondary schools shows why language disabled children are particularly at educational risk.

In primary schools increased awareness of children's language problems is beginning to lead to earlier identification of these children. Speech therapists, language unit teachers and psychologists are now alert to the possibility that primary school children may have language problems. Of course, resources are limited and there is considerable scope for in-service and pre-service teacher education about language difficulties, but in the primary school sector there is general recognition of the importance of language skills. There are many issues of assessment and teaching of reading and writing which remain controversial, especially since the publication of the 1988 Education Reform Bill, but there is a consensus that an important part of the work of the primary school is to teach children to read and write. Consequently primary school children with language problems are regarded as having difficulties with a key component of the school curriculum.

However, in secondary schools the situation is different. Little attention has been given to the difficulties faced by language disabled children when they are in secondary education. But research shows that problems with language will cause difficulties in most aspects of the secondary school curriculum (Beveridge & Conti-Ramsden, 1987). The central role of language in thinking and problem solving means that even apparently 'non-linguistic' subjects like maths and computing will be especially difficult for language impaired children.

At the present time, language disability is unlikely to be recognised as a cause of poor learning in secondary schools. And even if it were suspected, there would usually be little in the way of expert help and advice available. Most secondary schools do not have a co-ordinated approach to teaching language. Despite several initiatives, like the Schools Council 'Language in Use' Programme, it is still very unusual to find an operational policy for language across the curriculum.

Further, the approach to reading and writing in secondary schools differs from that in the primary sector, where literacy is part of the core curriculum. The secondary school system in England has, in recent years, been paying little attention to the explicit teaching and assessment of reading and writing. The assumption appears to be that the primary school has completed the task of teaching literacy skills. As a result, the secondary school English subject curriculum has been allowed to emphasise both 'creative writing' as an expressive art and the reading of literature as a route to understanding the rich and subtle nature of human lives. Other language skills are not being explicitly taught or assessed, with the result that schools have no formal knowledge of their children's level of literacy nor any systematic way of identifying the problems pupils have with reading and writing.

The recent Kingman report (DES, 1988) expressed deep concern with the general language skills of secondary school children, especially because of the importance of literacy in the education of older children. Reading and writing are necessary across the whole secondary school curriculum. Many school subjects require children to read and understand complex texts which are very different in nature from the narrative fiction encountered in the literature syllabus. A physics textbook makes very different demands on the reader from the poems of Philip Larkin. And writing an analytic piece about, for example, pollution for GCSE Geography is different from writing a narrative about a sea voyage.

Secondary school teachers are aware that some pupils do not succeed because of problems with literacy. But literacy is a controversial topic in many schools. It is not uncommon to find blame being placed on the English specialists for not teaching the literacy requirements of other subjects. For example, physics teachers will often complain that their pupils cannot write an experimental report and often regard the English department as responsible for their pupils' lack of language skill.

In fact English teachers have good reasons for being reluctant to teach language beyond its 'creative' role. They are concerned that teaching children about language will induce a 'mechanical' approach reminiscent of rote learning of grammar. By staying within the 'personal' and 'individual' aspects of the 'creative' arts, English teachers are able to foster a humanistic, subjective and interpersonal classroom atmosphere. This, they argue, does not turn children away from literature by presenting it as irrelevant to their own lives. Literature is used to foster awareness, expression of feelings and thoughts about complex human situations. Attempts to teach writing and reading for other purposes are seen by many English teachers as cutting across their central objective of bringing literature into the lives of children. They recognise the cross curricular demands for literacy, but resist systematic teaching of literacy on grounds which they see as relating to the core of the philosophy of English as a subject. Unfortunately, few teachers of other subjects typically have been trained in the analysis of language, and as a consequence are not fully equipped to tackle the problems of literacy. The situation in secondary schools will, therefore, be fraught with difficulties for the children who are less able to solve literacy problems on their own. Lack of support in literacy leaves them at great risk of failure within the secondary school system. And undoubtedly there are many children who are failing to achieve because of their low level of literacy associated with basic language difficulties.

A two-fold development is needed to help these children through secondary education. Firstly, a change of policy is required with respect to the teaching and assessment of literacy across the curriculum. A co-ordinated whole school approach to assessment and teaching of literacy skills is required across the school. And secondly, those children with difficulties in this area must receive diagnostic teaching which, at the earliest possible stage, prevents them being educational failures because of language difficulties.

It is not enough merely to bring this problem to the attention of those teachers concerned with language disabled children; the scale of the change required is too great. The crucial advance must be through a scheme for teaching literacy which provides a framework for both assessment and teaching. The first such nationally available scheme, Staged Assessments in Literacy (SAIL) has recently been developed and the remainder of the paper looks at this scheme and illustrates how it can help identify children with language difficulties.

One final point before outlining the scheme. Language difficulties are not independent of the demands that are placed on the language skills of children. The greater the demand the more likely problems will arise. The secondary school lays increasing emphasis on learning complex ideas through reading and writing. Hence many children who had previously shown no apparent difficulty with language may find their language skills are not sufficiently well developed to deal with the literacy tasks that school requires them to execute. Hence it is not only those children who have had language problems through their early childhood whom we have to consider, but also the problems which emerge for the first time in secondary school-aged children.

SAIL: A Framework for Reflecting on Written Language

Successful reading and writing requires children to integrate a number of different skills. They must also be ready to adjust their processing strategies during reading and writing. This requires that they are willing and able to reflect on their own reading and writing processes. Consequently children have to learn how to think about language and this is not a skill which comes naturally to them. The SAIL scheme recognises that many children will require help in learning to think about their writing and reading. It provides a way that pupils can direct their own reflections on the written word. The principles of the SAIL scheme apply to both reading and writing, but in somewhat different ways. The use of the scheme in helping children to write will be featured here, but a parallel application to reading is an important part of the complete SAIL programme.

The central problem children face in learning to produce satisfactory written text in secondary schools is knowing what it is they are supposed to be doing. When engaged in any writing activity the pupil is faced with a problem which is essentially one of communication. Pupils experience difficulty in clearly identifying the nature of the communication which is required. How do pupils know in what ways one writing task poses a problem which is different from another, or that a piece of writing which is effective in one context is ineffective in another? Pupils often have no systematic way of differentiating between the kinds of writing demanded by different tasks; when they read they tend to merely 'read', when they write they tend to just 'write'.

The literature on children's writing has clearly identified that novice writers use undifferentiated and unreflecting approaches (Scardamalia & Bereiter, 1983). They tend to respond to all writing tasks by saying anything that they happen to know about the topic. They fail to differentiate between the rhetorical purposes of different tasks. They tend to represent writing tasks in terms of the content rather than the type of communication required.

Teachers have an important role in weaning children away from this unreflecting and simplistic notion of writing which, as the SAIL approach points out, lacks the essential problem-solving feature of advanced writing. Teachers have to demonstrate to children that improvement in writing comes from making strategically appropriate decisions about the nature of the communication in which they are engaged.

When teachers set written activities which are new to the children they often fail to indicate that the writing required is a specific type, or genre, of communication. The children may even be unaware that there are generic forms of writing. The SAIL scheme, which is outlined in the next section, is designed to help children learn to write more easily, by identifying the types of writing which are required of them. Teachers can assist pupils to develop competence in writing by linking their written tasks to an overall approach to language. SAIL makes this possible by adopting writing type as a basis for a language syllabus. Language activities can be identified as belonging to conventional ways of communicating and specific strategies can be highlighted.

There has been a tendency for those working with language disabled children to concentrate on their difficulties at the sound, word and sentence level. These problems are very important but the central point made here is that we should not assume that reading and writing are best taught without reference to the communicative purpose which they serve; nor should higher level textual skills be neglected because children still have, for example, spelling problems or difficulties with sentence grammar. Furthermore, as already noted, secondary education demands high level textual skills which are not often formally taught. It is children with language difficulties who will benefit most from the explicit teaching of literacy. Also, we as practitioners will learn more about the difficulties that secondary school children have with language if we directly address the problem of teaching them the appropriate skills. Children, like those illustrated earlier, who have not been identified as having language problems, will be more likely to be seen as needing help. This difficult educational task requires a greater general understanding of the way language is put into written form to satisfy specific purposes. The remainder of this chapter illustrates, by outlining the SAIL language framework, the hidden complexity which faces both teachers and pupils in learning about written communication.

The SAIL scheme identifies fourteen different types of writing which commonly occur in school. These are shown in Table 1 together with the six stages of difficulty which are identified by the SAIL language framework. As an illustration of the SAIL approach Table 2 shows how one topic 'Styles of Clothing' can be the content of several different types of writing. This is, of course, what happens in the school context. Children cannot know which type of writing is required merely from knowing the content. They must also understand the language requirements. The important feature of the SAIL approach is that it gives children a framework which reveals the similarities and differences between types of writing. This gives them a systematic way of thinking about their writing. The scheme is also progressive in that it provides an ordering of difficulty of text types on which to base a teaching programme.

It is not possible here to discuss the whole scheme. I will consequently attempt to indicate what the scheme does, rather than how the individual components of language fit together so as to show children how to produce text. The detailed description is available in the SAIL handbook (1987).

TABLE 1 *This shows how the fourteen types of writing are organised into six stages within the SAIL scheme. The school subject areas in which these writing types typically occur are also shown*

	A guide to the stages	
Stages	*What you have to do*	*Subject areas*
Stage 1	*Personal account* Write about an occasion in which you have taken part. Show the order in which the activities happened.	All subjects
Stage 2	*Report* Write an objective account of an incident or activity. State clearly what happened and present the events in an ordered time sequence.	All subjects
	Imaginative account Imagine you are someone else and write a chronological account of your activities in such a way as to convey the imagined situation.	English History Geography RE/PSE
Stage 3	*Instruction* Write an orderly sequence of instructions which direct a reader towards a particular goal.	English Science CDT
	Explanation Provide an objective explanation through the use of examples and illustrations of how or why changes occur or how mechanisms work.	Geography Science CDT RE/PSE
	Description Write a detailed and factual description, grouping together similar features and characteristics.	All subjects

TABLE 1 *Continued*

Stages	*What you have to do*	*Subject areas*
Stage 4	*Opinion* Present a personal point of view by expressing opinions and giving reasons and/or examples to support them.	All subjects
	Narrative Write a story with a clear plot and characterisation. Manipulate the sequence of events for effect.	English
	Information Provide factual information about a subject, grouping together similar characteristics and covering particular aspects in detail.	History Geography Science CDT RE/PSE
Stage 5	*Compare and contrast* Set out the similarities and differences between two or more subjects ensuring a balanced and objective treatment of each.	English Geography History RE/PSE
	Reflection Through the expression of thoughts and feelings explore your personal response to an experience.	English RE/PSE
	Persuasion Attempt to influence a reader by recommending a particular belief or course of action.	English History RE/PSE
Stage 6	*Argument* Write an argument in which the basic premise is supported by sufficient evidence to make a convincing case.	English Geography History RE/PSE
	Analysis Consider an issue and evaluate conflicting evidence in an impartial and objective manner.	All subjects

TABLE 2 *This shows how the SAIL scheme can ask children to produce different types of writing about one topic. The example given is 'Styles of Clothing' which shows how one topic can be used as a basis for a writing task at all six stages*

Topic	*Styles of clothing*

Stage One: Personal Account

Choosing clothes can be difficult. How difficult it is depends partly upon who you are with at the time. Give an account of the last time you went shopping for clothes. Say where you went, who you were with and what you did.

Stage Two: Report

In a large fashion store an angry customer has made a complaint against a sales assistant. The floor manager has been called to the scene. You have witnessed all the events leading up to this incident. Write a report of what you saw stating precisely what happened.

Stage Three: Description

Teenagers of today choose between a number of quite different styles of dress. Select one teenage group and describe their dress. Give sufficient detail to allow an adult to recognise members of the group in the street.

Stage Four: Narrative

A young designer has just completed a collection of clothes for a fashion show. On the eve of the show a rival designer, known to be ruthless, pays a visit. Continue the story.

Stage Five: Compare & Contrast

Britain is a multi-cultural society. Select two cultural groups which have similarities and differences in their typical styles of dress. Compare and contrast the dress styles of the two groups.

Stage Six: Analysis

In some places of work such as schools, hospitals and prisons people are required to wear a uniform. Enforcing uniformity of dress, however, causes much debate. Consider this issue.

Within the SAIL scheme there are three keys to thinking about writing. These are the Focus, Use and Organisation of each writing type. Focus emphasises the reader/writer relationship. Research has shown that maintaining an appropriate relationship between reader and writer is an important component of writing skill. This feature of writing directs the writer's aim towards the producer, the audience or the content. The SAIL scheme refers to the different reader/writer relationships as writer, reader, and subject focus.

In writer focus the writing is used as a vehicle of expression to represent the writer's personal viewpoint. Information is selected to promote the writer's concerns, for example, when writing about one's own opinions, the writer's own views and experiences will be highlighted. Alternatively, when writing places the focus on the content, for example, in descriptive and explanatory writing, the emphasis will be on the topic. The third focus available to a writer is designed to influence the reader's behaviour or beliefs. Within the SAIL scheme this is termed 'reader focus'.

The second component of the SAIL writing framework concerns the use of information. Content can be used in three different ways: (a) to specify, which adds detail; (b) to expand, which clarifies relationships and (c) to examine, which evaluates information.

Writing tasks which require pupils to use information to specify, as when writing a factual description, personal account or instruction, use language to define or particularise. Clarity of expression and preciseness of vocabulary are particularly important. Alternatively, when information is used to expand, as when writing a narrative or exposition, children are required to give reasons or illustrations to support the content. The final way of using information, examining the content, is crucial for writing which is analytic or reflective in nature.

The third component of the SAIL framework is that of organisation: this refers to the principle used to order information in a written text. Several approaches to text description have identified the importance of the chronological features of ordering a text (Kress, 1982; Perera, 1984). Non-chronological text types have been identified as having either spatial or logical features (Wilkinson, 1986). The SAIL scheme identifies three ways of organising text: Time, Group and Theme. When producing texts ordered by time pupils organise their writing by presenting material with reference to the order of events as they occurred. It may not be that events are referred to in direct chronological sequence. Narrative, for example, may manipulate the order of events so as to keep the reader interested and explanation may introduce effects before causes. However the underlying ordering principle remains that of time.

TABLE 3 *This shows how the SAIL writing framework of FOCUS, USE and ORGANISATION relates to the fourteen writing types and the six stages*

Stage	*Type of Writing*	*Writing Focus*	*Content Use*	*Text Organisation*
1	Personal account	writer	specify	time
2	Report	subject	specify	time
	Imaginative account	writer	expand	time
3	Instruction	reader	specify	time
	Explanation	subject	expand	time
	Description	subject	specify	group
4	Opinion	writer	expand	theme
	Narrative	reader	expand	time
	Information	subject	expand	group
5	Persuasion	reader	expand	group
	Compare/contrast	subject	examine	group
	Reflection	writer	examine	theme
6	Argument	reader	examine	group
	Analysis	subject	examine	theme

Pupils are also often set writing tasks for which they need to organise by group. In writing about the history of weaponry or the emergence of medical care, it would be appropriate to organise text by putting the facts into related groups.

The third organising principle requires children to link material to one central theme. Analytical writing, for example, is best produced by bearing in mind a central idea which governs the decision to include and relate information. This idea will be identifiable as the theme of the text. It may appear in summary form in the text itself, or it may be there to be inferred by the reader. Its crucial feature is that it is represented organisationally.

The three dimensional framework just outlined is set out in Table 3. As spelled out in more detail, with examples, in the SAIL handbook, this writing framework is a means of helping pupils at all stages of the writing process. They are encouraged to use it in guiding their decision making from task analysis, through composition and revision. By applying the framework to different writing types they are acquiring, in effect, knowledge of different types of communication.

The full description of the scheme is available from the Joint Matriculation Board in the form of the SAIL Handbook. This shows how words, phrases, sentences and intersentential links relate to writing types. These features, as organised within SAIL, provide the language curriculum which is much needed in secondary schools, especially by those children for whom the current 'intuitive' approach does not work. Language disabled children are one such group and they must not be kept from literacy because teachers do not themselves understand how to communicate about types of text. As Beveridge & Conti-Ramsden (1987: 104) wrote

> . . . language disabled children can benefit from introducing literacy skills into their curriculum, and that even children with apparently severe sound/letter problems benefit from this 'top down' approach when it is combined with other methods.

However this will only happen in secondary schools when the general understanding of the structure and function of textual language is improved. Teachers will then be able to talk about the features of written text rather than concentrating on spelling and sentence grammar. This kind of help for the language disabled requires a radical shift in current educational practice with respect to language in secondary schools.

The SAIL handbook is available from the Secretary, Joint Matriculation Board, Manchester M15 6EU.

References

Beveridge, M. and Conti-Ramsden, G. 1987, *Children with Language Disabilities.* Milton Keynes: Open University Press.

DES (Department of Education and Science). 1988, *Report of the Committee of Inquiry into the Teaching of English Language.* London: HMSO (Kingman Report).

Kress, G. 1983, *Learning to Write.* London: Routledge and Kegan Paul.

Lee, A.D. and Shapiro -Fine, J. 1984, When a language problem is primary: secondary school strategies. In G.P. Wallach and K. Butler (eds), *Language Learning Disabilities in School Age Children.* London: Williams and Wilkins.

Perera, K. 1984, *Children's Writing and Reading.* Oxford: Blackwell.

SAIL Handbook 1987, Manchester: Joint Matriculation Board.

Scardamalia, M. and Bereiter, C. 1983, The development of evaluative, diagnostic and remedial capabilities in children's composing. In M. Martlew (ed.) *The Psychology of Written Language: a Development Approach.* London: Wiley.

Wilkinson, A.M. 1986, Argument as a primary act of mind. *Educational Review* 3, 2.

6 Structuring the curriculum in a language unit

ELLA HUTT

The Population of a Language Unit

The majority of the children in the ten special *schools* for the language handicapped in Great Britain have severe specific speech and language disorders. They are not caused by another handicap, such as low intelligence, hearing loss, or physical handicap. With most of the children the disorder occurs despite average intelligence, despite normal hearing, despite physical normality, and despite potentially normal ability to form social relationships. A minority do suffer from additional difficulties. But these are not so severe that the receptive or expressive language difficulties can be attributed primarily to them, so the language disorder is described as *specific*. We must, however, bear in mind that some aspects of each child's difficulty are less specific and/or less severe than others. This is even more true of the population of language *units*. In 1986, a questionnaire with a 50% response from teachers in language units in Great Britain, revealed that the types of language difficulties of their pupils could be described in fifty different ways. These descriptions can be reduced to a working list of nine, with many children having more than one difficulty:

(A) speech and language disorders in:

1. articulation
2. word-finding
3. phonology
4. expressive grammar
5. reception of speech
6. semantics
7. pragmatics of language

(B) 8. dysarthria

(C) 9. speech and language delay

Starting Points for the Construction of a Curriculum

It would be very surprising if all of these conditions, and a few more, were not encountered by staff in all language units. Many of them are faced with the problem of having to help children with as many different kinds of language difficulties as the number of children in their group.

So, how do they know where to start? And on what criteria do they base their decisions?

Most of these teachers are probably called upon to produce a curriculum which parallels that of the mainstream school in which their children are expected to work during some periods of the school week. But I suggest that this constraint is a matter of low priority. I further suggest that administrators who require this are asking for what is not only impossible, but also unfair to the children. Is it more important for a child to learn all aspects of language systematically, in the non-threatening environment of the language unit? Or should he be thrust prematurely into a classroom full of children of his own age who can do most things much better than he can? There he cannot fail to feel different, not only because of his lesser attainments, but also because he is required to be a member of two communities simultaneously. Many years ago, a nine-year-old boy from a special language school, with the least amount of language difficulty, was integrated twice weekly into the nearest primary school. All parties were co-operative, but all eventually realised that the venture was not a success. Now in his late twenties, this young man recently wrote:

> I have viewed the moves to integrate the education of the disabled with some scepticism, on the basis of my own experience. I am sure it is done with the best intentions.

There may be a few language units who are encouraged to create their own curriculum. But it would be good if more were allowed the freedom to experiment without the limitations imposed by mainstream needs and timetables. Not until a successful solution is reached should there be any kind of move to share lessons with mainstream classes.

Even when given this kind of freedom, where can one start? Many practitioners would say 'with language itself', meaning sounds and letters, words, meaning and grammar. Others would say 'with the foundations of language'. When a child first enters a language unit, are the foundations of language-learning not more important than the mechanics of word and sentence formation? The two-fold task of remediators is to provide opportunities for the expression of feelings and for real communication within the unit group; and to teach each child how to understand and use verbal language for these purposes. The priority aim subsumes the subsidiary aims of teaching him to attend and to concentrate; to understand the concept of representation; and to co-ordinate the parts of the body with each other, and with what he is thinking. It is the secondary aim which subsumes the mechanics of the understanding and use of language, in signing, in writing and reading, and in speaking.

So the priority aim at infant school level can be achieved by activities such as movement, music, drawing and painting, construction, and educational drama (see Figure 1). I have been sadly surprised by language unit teachers who have discouraged me from visiting their physical education session. 'It's only P.E.' is a remark I cannot understand. It is a subject too important to be dismissed. Even if language disordered children find P.E. and these other foundation activities difficult, their problems are unlikely to be as great as those they experience with language activities. Or, if they appear to fail when they are first introduced to music, painting or movement, they are likely to learn to enjoy it more quickly than the more formal aspects of language. One five-year-old boy with a severe receptive disorder hated joining in his first structured movement session. His response was to stand in the middle of the room and cry. But within a few weeks he was one of those who learned the sign for 'dancing', and used it as a frequent happy question.

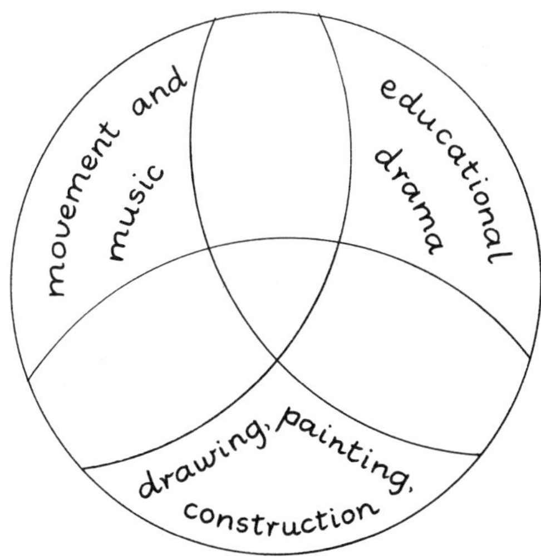

FIGURE 1 *Priority activities*

This anecdote illustrates the need to provide reasons for communicating. Many children learn to communicate well in spite of their spoken language problems. They use pointing and natural gestures which are quickly understood by those nearest to them. Some develop effective drawing strategies. A painting session often serves as a stimulus for a lot of conversation, as emerging works of art provide several common reference points. Construction activities, the corporate kind with boxes and paper, scissors and glue, lead to what might be termed discussion. And, in a group of children with less severe language difficulty, such a session often leads to exchange of information, about activities in the home and on holiday, seemingly irrelevant to the task in hand.

One of the commonest problems allied with what is described as a language difficulty, is that of not really grasping the concept of representation. Margaret Campkin quotes a child who asked, 'What "pretend" mean?' She introduced a variety of activities over a period of weeks. First the children experienced the reality of pulling the curtains, lifting a heavy box, and so on. Then they pretended to do them. The boy who had asked the question failed to get up from lying on the floor at the end of one lesson. The teacher thought he might have fallen asleep. But he was consciously pretending, and soon told her so. Children are encouraged to do individual imitations of others who are present, and similar ones later when the referents are absent. They can be led to work as teams, such as playing an imaginary, ball-less game of cricket. There are many types of representational and other activities which can be described as educational drama.

Music can be introduced in one or more forms: as a stimulus to painting or movement sessions. Music, like Holst's Jupiter or Mars, has helped to free some children's hands from clutching paintbrushes. Schubert's piano music is often used as the time-keeper for the structured exercises of Margaret Morris Movement. Dalcroze eurhythmics can be used to teach differences in the pitch, rhythm, speed, and other dynamics of music itself. Dr Ronald Senator's Musicolour Scheme has been adapted for use with language-disordered children. Children can learn to sing short simple tunes with a few memorable words, specially written to match a low level of comprehension and grammar. Games are played with percussion instruments or blocks of wood, to give practice in auditory discrimination.

The elements of Form Drawing, as used in Rudolf Steiner education, can be modified into activities for visual perception, imaginative thinking and hand–eye co-ordination, and for stimulating interesting conversation. A further good reason for concentrating first on the provision of what might be seen by some as purely 'fun' items, is that they are given proper consideration instead of appearing in the remediator's mind as frills. And, they can be tackled with a group, with no necessity for early pre-testing for setting individual goals. These can be set later, when subskills gradually become apparent.

Before embarking on any of these activities, it is not important to learn everything about a new approach. Experience with children with normal language can be put to good use. Teachers soon find out the ways in which a method has to be modified. It is not necessary to learn anything new to start with. They need to be clear in their own mind why they are doing each activity, and try not to allocate more than one specific aim at a time. Teachers must know what they are trying to achieve; be content if they do and not too pessimistic if they do not. They should let the children know when they are pleased with their efforts. And although these activities are not provided just for fun, this should always be there, as an unconditional bonus to teacher and pupil. At first sight it may appear logical that these activities could take place within mainstream classes. But this is neither practical nor kind, especially to a child whose language problem is a disorder, not a delay.

A Synoptic Consideration of Specific Language Elements

Since not every curriculum item can be introduced from the beginning, routines within these 'expressive representational' aspects can be established first. When general co-ordination improves, with it comes greater readiness for manual signing, writing and speaking. The representational construction through models or paintings of familiar objects, reinforces the concept of a sign or a word standing for an object, an action, or an attribute. At first the object should be visible but later absent, to encourage more advanced communication. (See Figure 2.)

It is the task of all staff in a language unit to take part in these activities, not just the teacher. When staff and children have got to know each other, then the appropriate time can be judged to introduce more difficult tasks: the manual signing of concepts, the recognition of whole words, and the handwriting of letters. These are gradually added within natural contexts.

Once a daily routine is established, a little more time can be spent in considering these further items, and the goals and methods for each. For example: is a manual sign system appropriate for the group of children for whom the unit provides? If it is necessary, for what purposes will it be

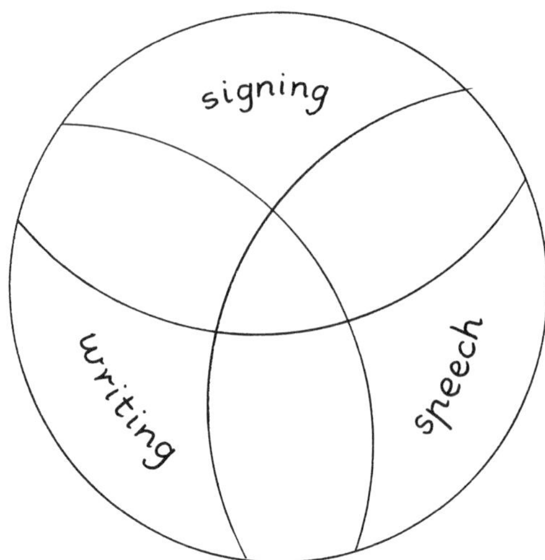

FIGURE 2 *Language learning media*

used? How many remediators will be willing and able to learn it? Only then can a realistic choice be made of a suitable system. Some comprise the kind of signs most suitable for basic communication; others, with additional signs for closed class words and word endings, are more suitable for the teaching of syntax and the other elements of grammar. Only a few systems are suitable for both. Some children need a manual sign system as an initial mediator between basic concepts and the corresponding written and spoken words in which they are expressed. Other children need to sign only when they are reading aloud, or only to accompany the words they cannot say intelligibly. The most useful systems, therefore, are those which can be adapted to a variety of needs.

The selection of a core vocabulary pulls the framework of the curriculum together. It is a reflection of the concepts which the remediators agree to teach. It is a time-consuming task, but ideally should be tackled before decisions are made regarding the choice of reading material and the purchase of supplementary word-based apparatus. How can children with limited or no spoken language be expected to learn to read from a series of booklets devised for children with normally developing spoken language? And sets of pictures should correlate with frequency of need. They should reflect the surroundings of the children in the school, and a selection of activities minimally beyond the school situation.

In the construction of a core-vocabulary, the most important items are the verbs and the closed-class words, that is, all words which cannot be classified as nouns or adjectives which are more likely to look after themselves. The more important verbs represent those actions in which all the children are likely to be involved. The sequence of closed-class words is based on the order of their inclusion in the syntactic strings to be taught.

The choice of schemes for the items which can obviously be labelled language-items follows the construction of a vocabulary. Handwriting can soon be incorporated into drawing sessions, and may even take so much time that for a few weeks very little drawing is done. This does not matter. It is one example of the way in which the time-table is altered to allow for temporary needs.

Detailed decisions must be made and carried out systematically. Schemes or sequences for spoken and written remediation should occupy a lot of discussion time between speech therapists and teachers. But it is time well-spent. The fewer the errors made during this co-operative exercise, the less time will be spent later in sorting out anomalies. Another vital decision, in which all must be involved, concerns the agreed methods of teaching spelling. And the problems of mathematics and thinking must eventually be faced.

Now that there are so many published schemes to choose from, it is very important that they should be chosen wisely in the first place, and used carefully according to the suggestions, for a realistic amount of time, before any similar scheme is considered as a replacement. There are many manual signing systems, many language-analyses, many language and reading programmes. There is an increasing number of handwriting, spelling and number schemes. But most of them have been devised for a particular group of special needs children or for handicapped adults. Their publishers do not usually claim that they are effective with other groups. Some do prove to be useful, but need more careful monitoring and adaptation than those which have evolved with a comparable population.

Curriculum Growth

A curriculum can never be considered finite. It is always growing. In a language school all members of staff can be responsible for searching out possible schemes, studying them and summarising the main features of each, so that comparatively quick comparisons can be made, followed by gradual curriculum decisions. But because there are fewer staff in a language unit, it may be more difficult to make such decisions. They cannot be made before the first children are known, and probably not even within the first term. Schemes not only have to be discovered, they have to

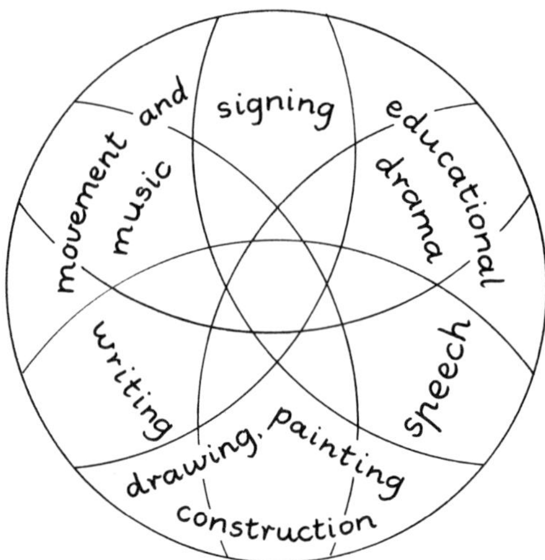

FIGURE 3 *A framework for a structured curriculum*

be learned, and, for many, some apparatus has to be made. It takes a long time for a new unit or a new teacher to become experienced enough in all the systems to feel at ease in their use. (See Figure 3.)

Gradually a curriculum framework becomes established, so that a new member of staff can be introduced to it without too much difficulty. The whole curriculum should be seen as an interlocking pattern. Depending on varying viewpoints of different observers, it may take on several patterns, like a kaleidoscope. One item may appear centrally to one person and on the fringe to another. But the pieces are contained, and always make a pattern. They also vary in importance for different children, at different stages, for different professionals, and on different occasions. But once an item becomes an accepted part of the curriculum, it is not likely to disappear. It is probable that the pattern may appear more complex with time, as additions and modifications are made. A remediator sees a particular need, and finds a way to meet that need, either by devising a new method on the spot, or by searching for one which fulfils her requirements.

Every scheme-user has to understand thoroughly the rationale behind it, so that he can judge when and where it is possible to alter an item, or omit it, or expand it. A teacher who asks advice from a colleague and then says 'Just tell me what to do. Don't tell me why' is not using a scheme responsibly. But it is also essential that one staff member should have a global view of all curriculum items being delivered at any one time.

She must know enough about every one of them to react wisely to suggestions about modifications, substitutions, or further innovations. She must recognise unnecessary redundancies and eliminate them on the grounds of economy, and bear in mind specific requests as she looks out for appropriate possibilities in other units with a similar population. She must be able to apply agreed criteria to others' suggestions, in order to give an informed opinion on their suitability in their situation. One scheme could be adopted as it stands, while another would need adapting first. For example, when confronted with a new maths scheme: does it include the vocabulary items which the teachers have decided are top priority? What proportion of the suggested activities are beyond the potential ability range of the unit? Does any page have more than one aim? Do numerals take precedence over basic concepts? Does the scheme go too far too fast?

Or, when looking at an unfamiliar reading scheme: does it progress according to a logical grammatical sequence? Does it depend too heavily on phonic ability in the early stages?

The Staffing of a Language Unit

It is essential that all the staff in a language unit are pursuing consistent goals. These must be implemented in a logically graded way, following as far as possible any suitable developmental stages. Each child's progress should be monitored, and although the rate of progress may not be regular, a definite sequence, developmental where possible, should be maintained. We are aiming to bring attainments in each aspect of the curriculum into line with all the others, to approach a better developmental balance. We follow a repetitive predictable routine, both within the school day, and within each curriculum item.

In order to meet the needs of the children, the professional staff in a unit for language-disordered children have to be curious, innovative and adaptable, with the minimum of preconceived ideas. At a recent conference, I heard two teachers discussing the ideas they had had about teaching language-disordered children before they had actually met any. One had experience in an infant school, and thought that language unit children would not be very different. The other had worked in a school for children with moderate learning difficulties, and thought that language unit children would certainly be very similar. They had both taught language. But they were shocked when they started in their units. The children were different, and so was the approach to language they had to employ.

Remediators have to put themselves in the place of the child, to try to understand what his difficulties really are. When a child cannot do something, what is preventing him: his poor attention or concentration, his limited perception, faulty memory, or his lack of co-ordination? Remediation requires recognition of the approximate place of breakdown, before help is given. Teachers need to acquire special teaching skills, which require application, determination and perseverance. This, in itself, provides an opportunity for a teacher to become part of a new learning situation. All the staff have to co-operate fully with other professional groups and to reach and tolerate necessary compromises. They have to accept an unpredictable mixture of pleasing and disappointing results. They should all be involved in the special curriculum: in devising and using it; in evaluating its parts and its cohesion; and perhaps modifying it, as the balance of needs change.

A structured curriculum, based on a consistent limited vocabulary, which combines the work of educational psychologists, therapists, teachers and assistants should be one of the main features of a unit for children with language difficulties, as should speech therapy. A curriculum has to be flexible enough to be followed at different rates of progress, and with different emphases, with children in the same unit class. Unit staff need clear descriptions of the type of language difficulties which will be accepted into the unit, so that the curriculum can be created from the beginning, in the most appropriate way. As it is such a complex task, it is important that selection criteria remain the same for a suitable period of time. Static goals can be reached more efficiently than moving ones. This is not to say that after a few years the situation cannot be thoroughly reconsidered, and modified arrangements made, but not after a few months.

Conclusion

An H.M.I., writing in the *Times* newspaper in 1901, gives us yet another general reason for allocating proper time to artistic appreciation and expression (Barnet, 1901). He suggested 'cultivating a rational power of enjoying beautiful things'. The expression of this is admiration. You must have met language-disordered children with an enormous capacity to appreciate. 'Look at that tree', said a seven-year-old boy who was totally enthralled by the sight of a tree in full blossom. Another, gazing at a drop of blood on a microscope slide, was full of amazement that it had come from his own finger. Now in his twenties, one of his main interests is astronomy. A well-planned project on a local coal-fired power-station resulted not only in a healthy respect for electricity, but also in a real sense of wonder about its production. Some of the happiest moments of language-disordered children have been observed when they are making things — cane-baskets, clay pots and aprons; collages and models; paintings and drawings; and plays.

To return to the H.M.I. — 'The teacher must do everything he can to place his pupils at the producers' point of view.' It is interesting that he concludes, 'Not until then should we ask them to examine the laws which lie at the surface of these things'.

Can't we say something similar about helping language-disordered children to learn language? Encourage them to produce their own art, and to appreciate others' productions. And, as this leads them to become more interested in communication, give them more information about learning the mechanics of language, and continuing opportunities to practise it.

Bibliography

BARNET, P.A. 1901, *The Times,* 3.1.1901, p. 5.

CAMPKIN, M. 1987, *Musicolour.* London: ICAN.

— (In preparation), *Educational Drama.* London: Invalid Children's Aid Nationwide (ICAN), 198 City Road, London, EC1V 2PH.

HUTT, E. 1986, *Teaching Language-disordered Children: A Structured Curriculum.* London: Edward Arnold.

HUTT, E. and DONLAN, C. 1987, *Adequate Provision? A Survey of Language Units.* London: ICAN.

NIEDERHAUSER, H.R. and FROHLICH, M. 1974, *Form Drawing.* New York: Rudolf Steiner School.

VANDERSPAR, E. 1985, *Dalcroze Handbook: Principles and Guidelines for Teaching Eurhythmics.* London: The Dalcroze Society, 26 Bullfinch Road, Selsdon Vale, South Croydon, CR2 8PW.

WHITE, J.W. 1980, *A Prophet Without Honour.* Glasgow: Margaret Morris Movement Therapy, Suite 3/4, 39 Hope Street, Glasgow, G2 6AG.

7 Patterns of mathematical learning associated with language disorder

CHRIS DONLAN

Widespread concern about levels of attainment in mathematics is nothing new, but it may be that the arguments have polarised recently. The 'back to basics' attitude has been central to Thatcherite educational policy and now enjoys considerable popular following. The educational establishment has for the most part been defending a broad approach to mathematics, and has firmly opposed government proposals for early and repeated 11-plus-type testing. Neither side can win this sort of battle outright. Recently it seemed that the Minister for Education was giving a little ground to the educationalists. But while the argument rambles on, pressure builds up on the teachers, at all levels in the education system. They are aware that they are expected to increase mathematical attainments but they are not necessarily sure how this can be achieved. Should they side with the educationalists and recognise the significance of mathematical language and go for more problem solving in the classroom, or should they give up what might seem an uneven struggle and return to rote-learning?

As is often the case, it takes children with language disorders to put the issues into clear perspective. For a long time we have been told that it is the 'language of mathematics' that is so vital yet so problematic. It is probably from this idea that schemes of mathematics developed which included instructions such as 'partition the set' to accompany tasks which might otherwise have appeared obvious. In retrospect it seems that an attempt was made to teach the scientific language of academic mathematics to young children. The certain knowledge that a young child with impaired language can do without that kind of help, clarifies the situation. For these children the phrase 'mathematical language' needs a less ambitious definition.

I suggest the following commonsense description of what is meant by mathematical language.

(1) The decimal number system itself.

(2) The use of numerical and relational terms in verbal communication.
(This is a vast uncharted area. It is not really a specialist area, simply that section of normal day-to-day verbal interaction which includes numerical and relational terms.)

(3) The use of abstract mathematical symbols to express relations between numbers.
(This is a specialist field. It includes Einstein's formulations of the Relativity Theory, but also the symbols used in simple arithmetic — the traditional base for early maths teaching and learning.)

Looking at mathematical language under these three headings can help us to organise our understanding of the learner's needs. It is clear that combinations of these components are required to perform practical day-to-day tasks. Shopping, for instance, may require a combination of all three components but it may be that most practical applications of maths, at least for the younger child, are covered by sections one and two.

We, in the adult population, have little enough confidence in our mathematical abilities. Martin Hughes, in a recent book (1986) notes that a team, commissioned by the Cockcroft Committee to research adult numeracy, found that half their sample refused to be interviewed simply because they were frightened of mathematics. How early is it in childhood that this kind of fear is born? Is the language-disordered child especially vulnerable to a mathematical phobia of severe and handicapping proportions?

The educational needs of children with a diagnosed language disorder are most commonly provided for either in special schools for the language handicapped or language units. The presenting problems tend to be more severe in the special school than in the unit setting. However there is considerable variation in the criteria for entrance to such provision, resulting in substantial overlap between the two populations — that is, between the children in special language schools and those in language units. Similarly the distinction between children in language units, in special needs groups, and those with special needs in ordinary classes, may not be clearly defined. This last group represents a large and diverse population which may have language difficulties similar in type to those more severe and specific problems found in special educational provision. The descriptions and examples given below are drawn from specialised settings, but they may be of relevance to some of the problems found in mainstream classes.

Language disorders are anything but uniform. It is more difficult to detect problems affecting a child's understanding of speech and language, but receptive difficulties often accompany the more obvious expressive problems. It is also possible for expressive difficulties to occur despite relatively intact receptive skills. Children with language disorders have usually been considered to have average non-verbal abilities — but this does not suggest that cognitive processes (at some level) are unaffected by this disability. The distinction between language and thought or processing capacity is slightly artificial here. Most children with language disorders present a complex profile, combining problems at different levels of the communication process. Possibly there can even be a sort of compensation effect whereby weakness, e.g. in the construction of meaning at sentence level, may be accompanied by strength in phonology. Furthermore, it is common for problems in language to be accompanied by difficulties in other domains e.g. in the perception and processing of visual information and problems in motor planning and organisation.

Given this complexity, we can hardly be surprised if, as Grauberg (1986) has pointed out, for language disordered children, 'There is no straightforward relation between (the degree of) language handicap and their difficulties in mathematics'. For this reason I want to make a strong plea for individual assessment of mathematical learning. I believe that if we are to tackle this very difficult and important curriculum area at all, we have to commit two of our most precious resources to it: those of time and thought. Time is never freely available but half an hour spent with one child, for whom maths is particularly difficult, would be a practical start. Thought is at times even more precious since a teacher's attention is drawn in so many different directions. However, thought is going to be necessary if we are going to deal effectively with this complex problem.

I want to suggest a framework for assessment. Obviously we must consider the special aspects of language appropriate to our client group and our subject area but we also need to look at the child's mathematical functioning outside a linguistic context. It is necessary to examine three areas of mathematical learning:

(A) the number system itself;

(B) non-verbal information processing;

(C) relational and numerical terms in verbal communication.

Within each of these categories, naturally, there is a progression or development. For the child beginning school these areas are sufficient in themselves. At a later stage it will be necessary to consider carefully the further category of formal mathematical symbols.

Degree of attainment compared across these different areas can be highly variable. Let us look at some examples (see Figure 1).

Two eight-year-old boys in a school for language disordered children were given a maths test, some items of which could be included under categories (A), (B), (C) as shown in Figure 1.

	Number system (A)		Non-verbal info. processing (B)		Relation & number terms in verbal comm. (C)	
	Pairs of numbers to 100 'Which is bigger?' (Verbal presentation)	Filling in blank 100 square	Grading Rods (e.g. Cuisenaire)	Seriation task, using given units to construct a seriated set	'Tell me 2 numbers that make x.' (Number Bonds to 10)	Count and find Xp. (Understanding composite units of money)
M. 8;1						
R. 7;9						

FIGURE 1 *Schematic representation of results obtained from a mathematics test given to two eight-year-old language disordered boys. Shading represents an estimate of degree of success.*

These two examples have been chosen because they are highly contrastive. M. has specific phonological problems, largely uncomplicated by difficulty at other levels of language. He has trouble with the number system itself. It is clear that poor speech perception and production presents an extra barrier in learning the already unsystematic sound/

symbol correspondences in the decimal system. As far as reasoning is concerned M. is fine. He actually performed the seriation task using an x + 1 principle, the only child in his class of nine to do so. He is able to cope with verbal discussion of number bonds, and is starting to deal with composite units of money according to verbal instruction.

R. shows the opposite profile. He is able to cope perfectly with the 100 square and even the 'bigger number' question. He is able to perform the grading task but does not notice missing steps and is unsure where the missing items should be inserted. The items in C are quite beyond R's reach. The nature of R's language problem is quite different from M's. He is strong phonologically, but has problems at the syntactic and semantic levels: he is hesitant in conversation, has poor control of context and content, and has additional difficulties in motor organisation. His mathematics profile is potentially more misleading than M's. His fluency with the number system conceals a poor processing ability and considerable deficit in practical mathematical communication.

Now let us look at some younger children; six- and seven-year-olds in a language unit. The tasks are at an earlier stage, but fall easily into our categories A/B/C (Figure 2).

D. shows a similar profile, and similar language problems, to R. (Figure 1). K. and S. have phonological difficulties. S. shows an additional comprehension problem. These characteristics of the children's language difficulties are directly reflected in their mathematical profiles. This sort of information is useful for developing teaching strategies. The speech therapist may be able to advise on appropriate teaching to help K. and S. with their number systems, and we can certainly look to provide visual support, e.g. Cuisenaire rods/Eva Grauberg's quantity pictures (Grauberg, 1985). In D's case teaching strategies need to point in quite a different direction. It may be most useful here to look at early cardinal values, and very carefully relate this to practical sorting work. The verbal negotiation of quantity and measure require a specially careful approach. P. proved to be a very special case. His very severe comprehension and expressive difficulties require him to use signs to communicate. Despite this, his visual 'thinking' is evident, his grasp of the number system is developing, and his computational skills are good. P's need is very much in area C where the mathematical skills he possesses must very gradually be put into a communicative context.

I have tried to emphasise the importance of looking at mathematical learning in terms of categories or areas which I believe to be helpful when assessing the language impaired learner. I have chosen specific, simple,

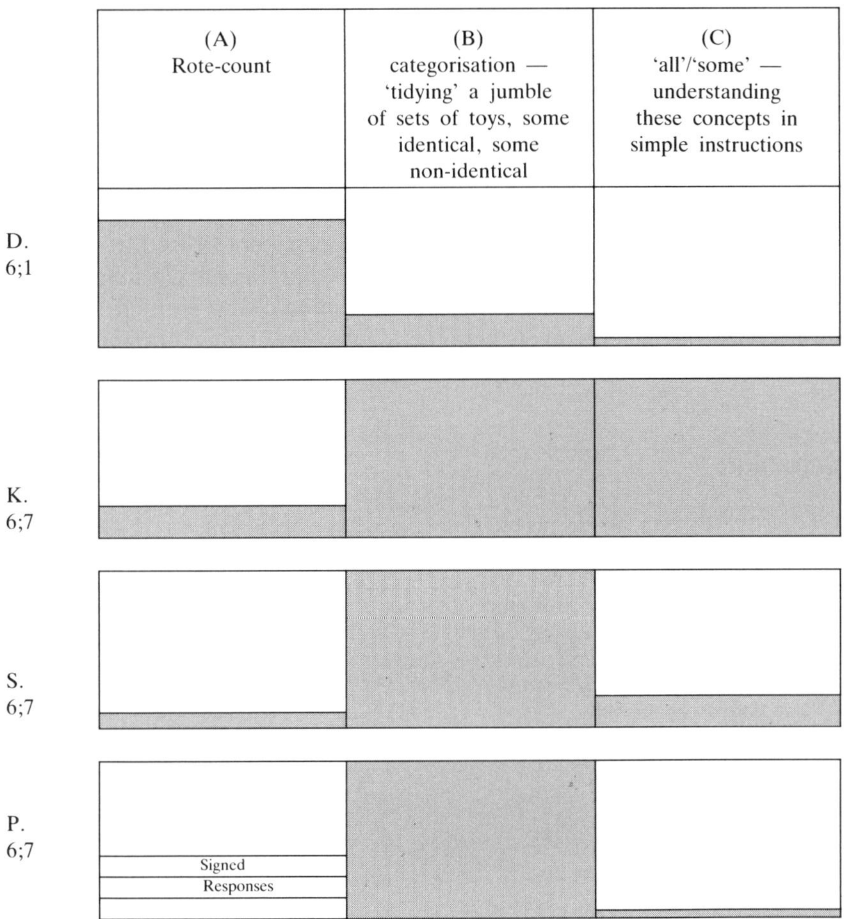

FIGURE 2 *Schematic representation of results of mathematics tasks given to six- and seven-year-olds in a language unit*

and easily explained examples to illustrate contrastive learning patterns. Clearly, assessment cannot depend on the few tasks I have mentioned. Each learning area must include a progression of tasks of developing complexity, having some sort of consistency across categories, and including, eventually, a section dealing with formal mathematical symbols. Work in progress for the charity ICAN aims to produce such a procedure, for the 5–8 year age-group (Hutt & Donlan, work in progress). It is hoped that a structured assessment procedure, for identifying group and individual needs will allow professionals to apply their skills more effectively. Given a clear identification of goals, there is every reason to employ teaching strategies which have proved to be appropriate for language impaired learners across the wider curriculum. Visual methods have proven value (e.g. Cuisenaire rods, Paget Gorman Signed Speech, Grauberg's 'Paper Abacus'); small group games are useful for developing communicative skills; child-centred content is crucial and a structured programme in the teacher's mind makes for effective learning by the children. It is hoped that the Mathematics Assessment Procedure, soon to be available, will itself provide a structure for mathematical teaching for the early years of schooling. A realistic definition of the problem will help us not only to cope effectively with the teaching of mathematics but also to enjoy it.

References

GRAUBERG, E. 1985, Some problems in the early stages of teaching numbers to language-handicapped children. *Child Language Teaching and Therapy* I.1., 17–29.

— 1986, Feeling at home with number symbols: some suggestions for the teaching of numbers to language-disabled children. *Advances in Working with Language Disordered Children*. London: ICAN.

HUGHES, M. 1986, *Children and Number Difficulties in Learning Mathematics*. Oxford: Blackwell.

HUTT, E. and DONLAN, C. (work in progress), *M.A.P.–Mathematics Assessment Procedure for Young Language-Impaired Children*. London: ICAN.

8 The parents' role in supporting children in education

RICHARD DA COSTA

My short paper concerns the role of the parent, and I hope to give you a feel for how educationalists and parents can work together to the benefit of language disordered children.

I write as a parent of three children, two of whom attend a special school as a result of a speech and language handicap.

It is now accepted practice that by assembling a group of multi-disciplined professionals and adopting a 'team' approach to the management of children with special needs, it is possible to achieve the necessary specialist input yielding maximum gain to the child. I would like to propose that the role of the parent in this situation is to be a pro-active and participative member of this team.

Let me straight away add that in no way would I, as a parent, seek to usurp the skills of the professional, but it is my belief that in the field of special educational needs, of which I have experience, the professionals and the parents are mutually interdependent.

In particular, I wish to propose five key aspects of the parents' role to develop this idea, and these are:

–The supportive role
–The communicative role
–The role of security provider
–The stimulating and developing role
–The re-inforcement role.

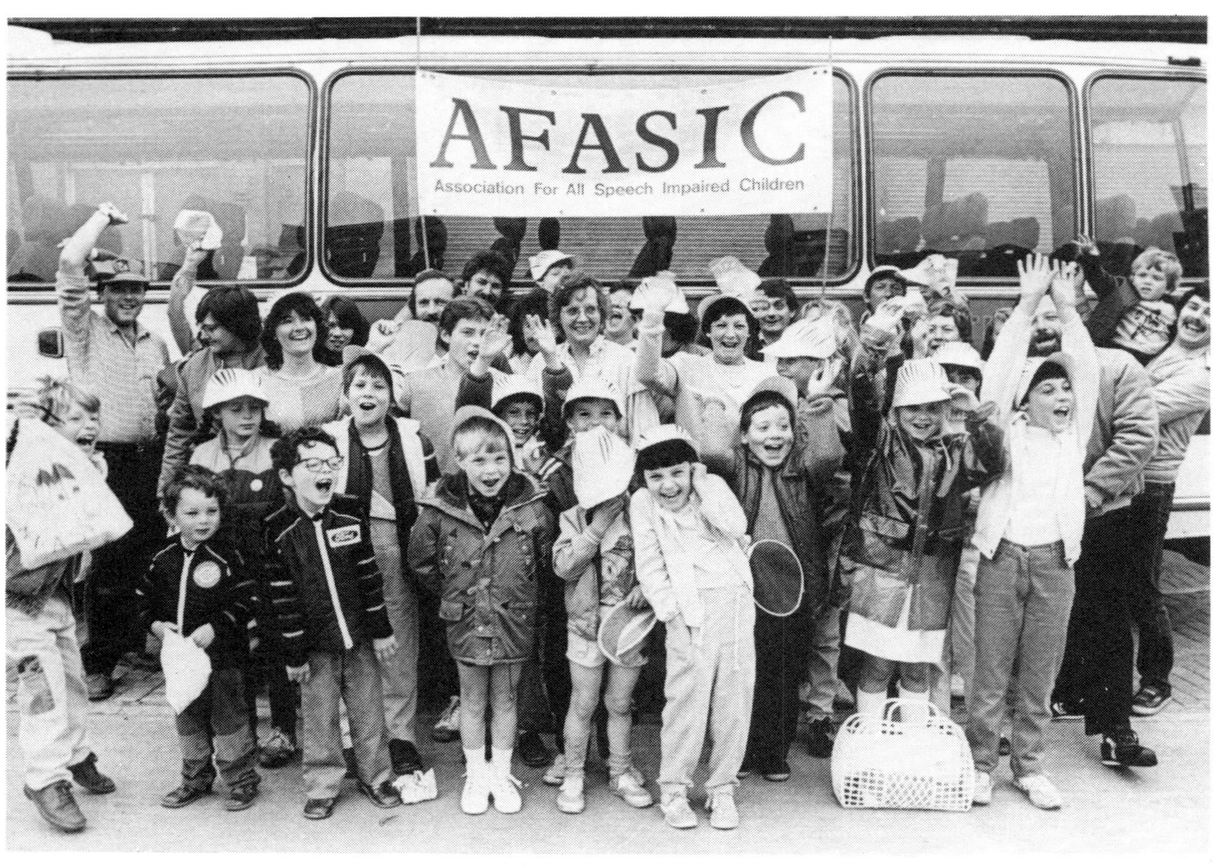

Parents and children enjoy a stimulating day out together.

The Supportive Role

There are two aspects to this topic. There is the need to support the efforts of your child, something all parents do whether their child is handicapped or not. There is also the paramount need to support the efforts of the teacher and/or therapist.

Now this is where I lapse into writing from personal experience, which is a most useful device when I do not want to be in fear of contradiction.

So, personal experience in this context has shown that our children are not persistent in the classroom; they give up far more readily than non-speech-impaired children. If we support the efforts of the child we are most likely to achieve success, but if we are seen by the child to support the efforts of the teacher, then this is a powerful message which will gradually boost confidence and lower resistance.

Eventually, it is to be hoped that behaviour adopted at school becomes the norm at home and/or vice versa, and all the good work is not undone by parents failing to support teachers and just as importantly teachers failing to support parents.

Let me digress for a brief moment to make a point. I implore educators to recognise please, that just as you have educational goals and objectives for our children, so we as parents have goals and objectives and certain values that are important to us. Hence the way for you to obtain our support, and you need it, is to consider ways to support us at times.

The Communicative Role

You would expect this role to be important when dealing with a speech and language handicap, but how often do we truly communicate? Again my main theme here is the communication between parent and teacher. This is particularly so in those first formative one or two years at school.

The pressure and anxiety a child can experience at school is well known. It seemed to take our boys nearly two years to settle. School is initially unnatural, particularly the relatively intensive concentration required compared to probably very little if any prior to school. If we accept this premise, then it must be in all our interests to have children relax as soon as possible. The way to do this, surely, is again for the child to see that the teacher actually communicates with his or her parents.

In other words there is a real link between school and home, not just a once a year parental visit but meaningful communication concerning the child's habits, interests and domestic activities which can become part of school routine. This will clearly demonstrate to the child that school and home are part of a continuum, and not, as we so often see, two separate activities specifically designed for children to set in motion against each other! (aren't they clever at doing so even if they can't talk?).

There is, of course, no doubting the importance of school and school life in the educational and social development of children. Children with special needs often have a greater social handicap enforced upon them by the isolation that a language unit or special school can create.

Now this is not the time or place to join the great integration debate, but if we all concentrate on the communication process between us as teachers and parents, then there is a much greater chance that the risk of inhibiting social development will be minimised through general awareness and acceptance of the problem.

Finally, I believe that the responsibility for this communication lies jointly with the parent and the teacher and that we must help each other with this. After all we surely cannot be guilty of the very thing that brought us together, lack of communication.

The Role of Security Provider

Despite the fact that we are probably the only animal species who send their offspring away from the family to be educated, those same offspring still look to the family for security.

For how long a child will carry on looking for parental security will of course depend to a large extent on the individual, and this in turn will depend on the level of self confidence which exists within that individual to 'go it alone'.

In some of us, the urge for independence and the necessary assertive skills are strong and seemingly natural; in others they are acquired and developed by training or self discipline.

In some, and I revert again here to personal experience, self confidence is minimal and soon lost, and assertiveness is something others do to you.

I have seen our boys in unfamiliar surroundings or with strange people display what appear to me to be totally alien characteristics. They become quiet, shy and withdrawn. Indeed at one time, this behaviour was the norm anywhere outside home.

We have had to be hard and almost ruthless in forcing them to accept the unusual and the different. Our fear was that they would be too frightened to ever cross the threshold of the house and so we felt it was a case of being cruel to be kind.

I have no doubt that this approach is necessary, and I also have no doubt through talking to other parents in AFASIC that this lack of self confidence is all too common among children with a speech and language handicap.

Now the trouble with a lack of self confidence is that it is like a self fulfilling prophecy; the more you think about it, the worse it is.

The truth about this problem is that I do not know what the answer is, but what I do know is that it is and must be the job of parents to be absolutely certain that our children at least feel totally secure domestically and have the confidence to develop their characters at least within the confines of their own home.

There are many exercises and techniques which I use in business to develop assertiveness amongst managers, but I confess to being at a loss as to how to introduce these techniques to young children. For this I have to rely on teachers, but again it is the responsibility of the parents to support the teacher.

Remember security is a basic human need, and our children have enough problems without adding this to the list.

The Stimulating and Developing Role

This is obviously important to any child, but I think this role with a handicapped child is accentuated. This is because, being honest, the provision of stimulating events and activities usually requires more parental energy input than with non-handicapped children. It is therefore easier to put it off when just the thought of it wears you down!

Many are the times that my wife and I have suggested something simple to the boys, like going for a walk, and by the time we have explained three times over, in words of one syllable or less, where we are going, with whom, why, and so on, we are both too exhausted to set foot out of the door.

Now there are many non-handicapped hyperactive children who can wear the patience of Job thin, but with our children you know that they are like self-cleaning cassettes; it doesn't matter how many times you record the message it wipes itself clean as you go along. In other words effective memory is minimal.

What this means in early childhood is that the term 'parrot-fashion' takes on a whole new meaning. Every experience is new because the last time the child experienced it is beyond the effective memory span.

Again, the isolationist nature of special schools and units can mean that a whole range of social experiences are missed, and it is undoubtedly parental responsibility to try and provide these.

Because of this, the role of developer and stimulator takes on an extra significance, and leads neatly into my last parental role, that of the re-inforcer.

The Re-inforcement Role

You may have noticed that there are certain common themes running through most of what I have written so far. One of these common themes is the constant need to re-inforce.

At all times I suggest to you that it is vital for parents to know what is happening at school so that we may be supportive. Indeed, you could say that if parents and teachers learn to communicate effectively with each other and ensure the provision of psychological and physical security while developing and stimulating our children and constantly re-inforcing, then we have created the ideal educational environment to provide what our children lack.

Conclusion

Above all else, I think that the combination of these parental roles should come together to provide a stable and effective balance between the needs of a normal family coping with youth and its many forms of expression, and the special needs of treating a handicap.

We must never lose sight of the fact that these children are handicapped, but more importantly we must never forget that they are children. We can therefore take as normal, and in some cases be delighted to see it, a certain amount of mischief and misbehaviour.

It is the balance between this and over protection, over indulgence and lack of patience that we as parents are not prepared for.

However, just in case we do ever become too full of our own importance to our children, let me draw to a close by telling you an anecdote that demonstrates how all of our theories come tumbling down in the face of inescapable childhood logic, guaranteed to humble the most thoughtful parent, and I quote:

Child to Father (with fingers in mouth)	'Why are some teeth different to others?'
Father to Child (trying to awaken a ten-year-old's interest in biology)	'Well, some are sharp for cutting and they are called incisors and some are blunt but big for grinding and crushing and they are called molars.'

N.B. Note the communicative, developing and stimulating roles played by the father here!

Child to Father (instant response)	'Is that why we bury people when they die?'
Father to Child (trying desperately to re-inforce his idea but failing miserably to even understand it)	'EH??'
Child to Father (with supreme cerebral logic)	'So the moles can have our molars to dig holes.'

The moral of this is surely that the key role of the parent is undoubtedly to be the butt of infantile one-liners which defy all serious educational analysis.

Dear reader, you may or may not be any wiser now as to the role of the parent, but I thank you for your attention.

9 The work of the Association For All Speech Impaired Children

MOIRA NOBLE

AFASIC was founded in 1968 by Margaret Greene, a speech therapist, concerned that children with communication impairments and the needs of their parents were being largely ignored. The aim of AFASIC is —

> To promote the interest and the well-being of children and young adults with speech and language difficulties where this is their primary handicap.

Our aim has remained the same since 1968 although, because we are a dynamic organisation, there have inevitably been changes in the approaches we have adopted in order to achieve that aim.

The Association is organised around the Central Office staff based in central London — a small staff of six, one of whom is part-time. The Central Office staff service the membership of nearly 1800 who are organised into Regional Groups scattered throughout the country. There are currently 30 of these which are made up of our parent and professional members. It is important that we have a mixed membership. We are not solely a parent organisation, we are not solely a professional organisation. Our dual membership is reflected in the way in which we approach our work and in the type of projects in which we become involved.

Looking at our work, it can be divided into three general areas of activity. Firstly, we campaign for improved provision (i.e. the educational and employment prospects available to those with communication impairments).

Secondly, we promote awareness of communication impairments. We concentrate our energies on the general public, professionals who are not familiar with this rather specialist field, policy makers (who in the end decide what provision is available to our children and young people), and the service providers (those who at the local level, are responsible for ensuring that these children are managed effectively).

Thirdly, we provide services; we provide services for our parents, for professionals, and for the children and young people themselves.

I will now look more closely at each of those three areas and discuss in more detail what each aspect involves.

Campaigning for Improved Provision

There can be no question but that educational provision for our client group is inadequate. We estimate that there are 220,000 communication impaired children in Britain (this excludes those who have a mental handicap). This is the figure which we use to determine the level of provision to which our campaign must be directed. At the very least, we maintain that there should be one speech therapist for every 3000 of the school-age population. To achieve this, we would need to see a doubling or even trebling of speech therapy establishments. Furthermore, we would like speech therapy departments resourced in such a way as to enable therapy to be delivered as a matter of course to our children in an educational setting, allowing therapists and teachers to work together effectively.

The number of specialist teachers is also inadequate. For our estimated 220,000 children we need 38,000 trained teachers: 40 teachers completed the Reading University in-service training course which was established by AFASIC in 1979. Unfortunately, because of difficulties in securing year-long secondments from local education authorities, this course folded in 1986 leaving those wanting to work in this field to learn largely through experience. We were therefore delighted to hear of the opening in 1987 of a two-year part-time DAES course on Child Language and Language Disability for experienced teachers in the Department of Speech at Newcastle-upon-Tyne University. AFASIC runs occasional one-day workshops for language unit teachers and therapists, and the Invalid Children's Aid Nationwide (ICAN) is active in disseminating the expertise built up over many years at their specialist schools. But this is blatantly inadequate when 38,000 trained teachers are needed.

Another aspect we should not forget in this connection is the question of the career structure in which language unit teachers operate. We need to attract teachers of high calibre to enter this specialised field and we cannot expect to do so in any great numbers if the specialist skills they have to acquire and the degree of responsibility they take on is not rewarded.

At the moment there are only a handful of schools which cater for communication impaired children. There are only 200 language units, the majority of which cater for those under 11. We are very concerned that there is so little for secondary age pupils and absolutely nothing for those needing placement in further education. We need to see a substantial increase in the number of educational placements available — a doubling at the very least, and at least a beginning in further education.

Employment prospects for our young people are poor and this is something which causes us concern. We are having discussions with relevant organisations to establish what the need is in terms of training and employment schemes.

So, by campaigning for improved provision, I mean we work towards an increase in the number of speech therapists, the number of trained teachers and the number of specialist educational placements.

Our campaigning role involves lobbying central government, largely an information-giving process. We lobby MPs individually, whoever is appropriate at a given time, or when we discover a Member with an interest pertinent to our aims. We submit evidence to the House of Commons' Select Committees inquiring into issues with which we are concerned, for example, we were active in ensuring that the Select Committee examining the effectiveness of the 1981 Education Act was made aware of the needs of our children. We meet frequently with officials from the Department of Education and Science and the Department of Health and Social Security. Recently we held a joint meeting with both of those bodies to address the problem of speech therapy provision in the context of the 1981 Education Act. Generally, we seek to influence Central Government by focusing attention on our children.

At a local government level, we work to inform local education authorities and health authorities of the needs of our children. It is often through our Regional Groups that pressure is brought to bear at a local level through meetings and general lobbying. Individual case work which we take on at Central Office can result in increased provision generally in the area in which the case arises. We use the 1981 Education Act to insist that local education authorities make appropriate provision and by forcing the issue for a particular child we often bring about a change in the general policy pursued by the Authority, such as a move towards establishing language units.

While our campaigning work frequently involves us in putting pressure on authorities, we also pursue our aims by offering support. Our

Regional Groups are very active in raising money to equip language units, to fund speech therapy posts and to fund mobile speech therapy units, which encourages health and education authorities to improve provision.

Promoting Awareness of Communication Impairments

The second aspect of our work is to increase awareness of communication impairments. This is a goal in itself although obviously, it does have campaigning implications; the more people know about communication impairments, the easier it is to harness the support of the general public in pressurising policy makers and service providers to meet the needs of those so handicapped. Of course, the audience to which we direct our efforts goes beyond the 'general public', including policy-makers, service-providers and professionals who are not familiar with this area.

To give particular attention to the professional audience, we see raising awareness amongst this group as important in the context of our fight against mis-diagnosis. We do not expect every health visitor, educational psychologist, paediatrician, GP or teacher to be a specialist in communication disorders. Our aim rather is to make them aware of the danger signs so that they are able to quickly refer cases to the right professional. Our Speech and Language Problems Screening Test (SLPS) described by Corcoran in this volume, is designed to give mainstream teachers the guidance they need to make such referrals.

Increasing awareness of communication disorders improves the lives of our young people and their parents. A few years ago I met an 18-year-old girl, diagnosed at the age of five as language impaired. She had benefited from specialist teaching and therapy, and is now in full time employment; someone who has successfully overcome the major problems associated with the handicap. However, she thought her life would be easier if people understood her problem — if she were able to go into a shop and not be treated as though she were stupid. Parents often tell me that what makes it so much worse having a handicapped child, is the fact that their family and friends do not understand, and dismiss their attempts to explain as their failure to accept that their child 'isn't very bright' or is just badly behaved when a frustration tantrum is running its course.

And of course, explaining the nature of communication disorders is very important in the context of our fund raising activities; without an understanding of communication impairments, people are unwilling to donate to an organisation which represents those suffering from those

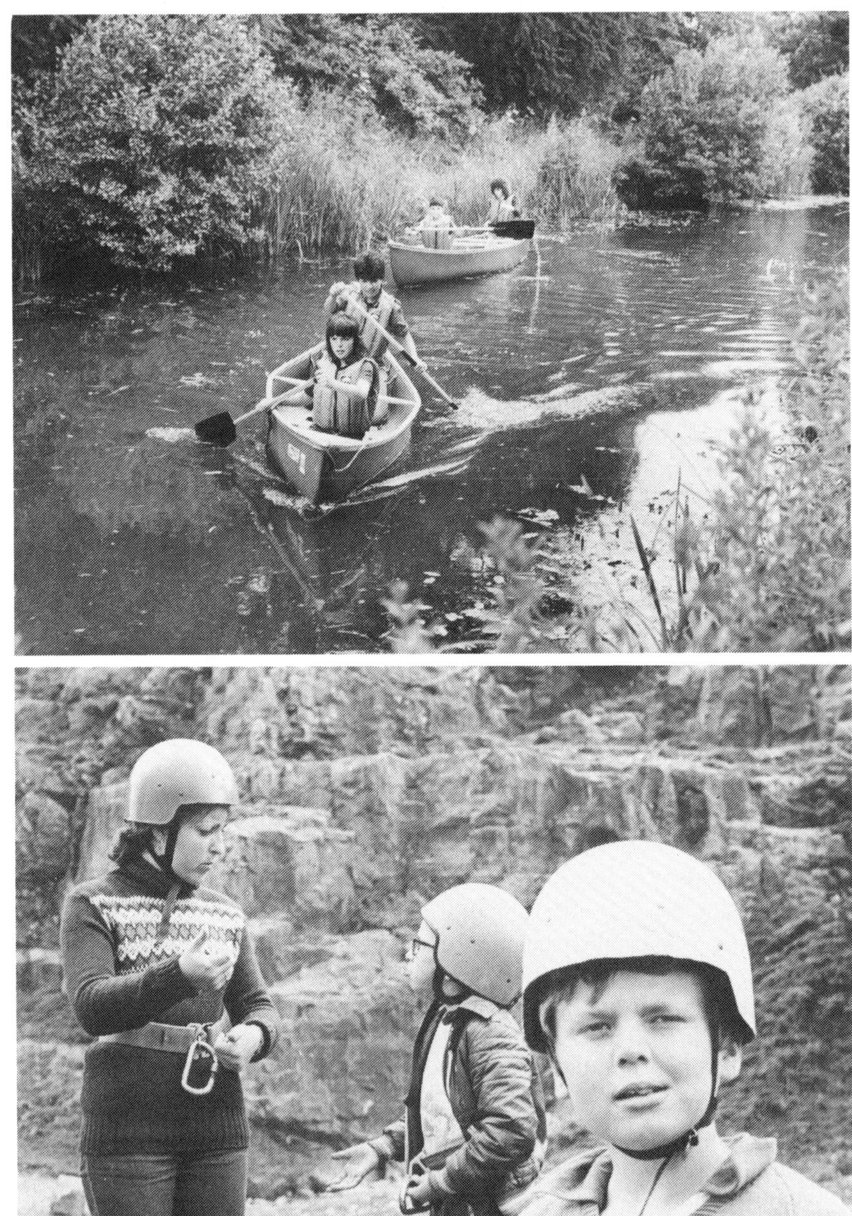

AFASIC Activity Weeks and Weekends offer challenging holidays with opportunities for self-development.

impairments, and then of course AFASIC could no longer continue its work.

The means by which we promote understanding is through our AFASIC literature, media attention and through the activities of our Regional Groups in their communities.

Providing Services

The third aspect of our work is service provision. We provide advice and support to parents through our Newsletters, published three times a year, and through our Regional Groups, where at the local level, there is the need for emotional and moral support. In addition, Central Office in London takes on individual case work, assisting parents involved in disputes, perhaps with education authorities or health authorities, or those trying to have assessments completed on their children.

We run Activity Weeks and Weekends for our children and young people throughout the year, offering challenging holidays with opportunities for self-development. These Activity Weeks were started with the needs of parents primarily in mind. Elizabeth Browning, our former Chairman, visited a parent many years ago and recalls trying to talk to this mother, a single parent, with a language impaired child in the room. The child kept interrupting and demanding the mother's attention, who was obviously reaching the end of her tether. Elizabeth Browning realised that the parent needed a rest, seeing it as AFASIC's responsibility to help the parent as much as the child, hence the first Activity Weeks/Weekends in 1972.

We provide advice and support to professionals working in this field. Our Newsletters inform them of courses, put them in touch with other professionals working in different research areas and report on new developments. Often we act as an information resource, responding to queries ranging from curriculum for language units to educational facilities, passing people on to appropriate sources of help.

Throughout the year we run workshops for teachers and speech therapists. We hope that an AFASIC initiated in-service, distance-taught course for teachers will soon begin at Birmingham University and Polytechnic, replacing the AFASIC Reading University course which closed in 1986.

Other aspects of interest to professionals are our research project in progress in West Berkshire which is examining diagnosis procedures, and the International Symposium in 1987. This proved so successful that it is to be repeated in 1991. The Symposium stimulated research and gave opportunities to research workers to present new and fresh material to their colleagues. The rare opportunity to exchange ideas gave further impetus to research which is desperately needed.

We provide services for the children and young people themselves. Our Activity Weeks/Weekends are extremely popular. In addition we have various projects going on throughout the year; including in 1988 a series of arts and crafts weekends for our children and young people; we have organised a Tall Ships voyage for a number of the older age-range.

This is a brief outline of the work of AFASIC. We are a dynamic organisation, constantly responding to the many new demands which are made on us. For example, current integration policies mean that mentally and physically handicapped children are now being taught in mainstream schools — their physical and learning difficulties are being accommodated so their communication problems are becoming more apparent, an issue which we must address.

Any media attention we receive leads to an expansion of our work as our membership increases. There are constant new demands being made on the organisation by our membership; there is always a call for more support. In particular, recently, we have become aware of a need to make professional counselling available to our members' older children on matters such as personal relationships and employment issues. Inevitably, the children of our early members are now grown up, and are in their 20's or 30's so it is time for us to really address the problems faced by adults and school-leavers with language impairments. Campaigning for language units alone is not enough.

Clearly, there is a tremendous need for more research in all areas connected with this subject. There are so many questions to ask about the nature of communication and about effective remediation when it breaks down.

So, these are some of the issues that we are looking at when we consider the expansion of our work. AFASIC, I am sure, given the support of our membership and the dedicated professionals who help us achieve our aims, will successfully meet these new challenges.

ANNOUNCEMENT

DEPARTMENT OF SPEECH
University of Newcastle upon Tyne

Two-Year Part-Time
DAES Course
for Experienced Teachers
(with BPhil option)
on Child Language and
Language Disability

Special arrangements made for out-of-district participants

For further information and application form, please write to:

Department of Speech
University of Newcastle upon Tyne
St Thomas Street
Newcastle upon Tyne NE1 7RU
Tel: (091) 232 8511

Index

Note: Numbers in italics refer to tables and figures; AFASIC = Association For All Speech Impaired Children

AFASIC
 –aim 90
 –campaigns for provision 91–3
 –organisation 90–1
 –promoting awareness 93–5
 –promoting services 95–6
 –screening-test development 31, 35–6, 93
American Psychiatric Association, Diagnostic and Statistical Manual 3–4
Articulation 12, 17, 22, 28, 65
Assessment
 –for mathematics 78–82
 –psychological 50
 –Staged Assessments in Literacy Project (SAIL) 51–2, 56–64 *see also* evaluation
Aston Index 26
Attention, problems of 5, 16
Audience, awareness of 62

Beveridge, M. 51–64
Beveridge, M. & Conti-Ramsden, G. 64
Birmingham
 –Primary Intervention Procedures 42–51
 –Visiting Teacher Service 41, 43, 49, 51
Bridgeman, E. 26
Browning, Elizabeth 1, 95

Campkin, Margaret 68
Carey, Susan 18
Chazan, M. 32
Cleft lip and palate, and reading problems 12, 23
Co-operation, professional 5–6, 29, 74
Communication
 –stimulation 68, 75
 –in writing 57–8
Competence, language 8–9, 20
Concept development 17–18, 19, *48*, 48
Construction, importance in curriculum 67–8
Conversation, incidential 45
Corcoran, Joanne 2, 31–9
Cruttenden, A. 14, 17
Crystal, D. 32
Curriculum
 –language unit
  growth 71–3
  specific elements 69–71
  structuring 66–9, 74
 –theme-based 42, 46

Da Costa, R. 83–9
Delay, language 3, 24, 66
Development, cognitive 17, 78
Development, language
 –school children, 8–10
  and child development 9–10
  language levels 11–20
 –variation 31–2
Discourse 13
Discrimination, auditory 26, 27, 68
Disorder, developmental 4
Donlan, Chris 76–82
Drama, importance in curriculum 67–8
Drawing and painting
 –Form Drawing 68
 –importance in curriculum 67–8, 71
Dysarthria 65
Dyslexia
 –and articulation problems 22
 –and literacy 24
 –phonological 28

Dysphasia, developmental, *see* language impairment, specific
Dyspraxia, developmental verbal, and reading and spelling problems 22–3, 25–7

Education
–further, provision 92
–mainstream
and needs of language impaired 2, 33, 41, 43, 67, 96
numbers of language impaired 40–1
Education Act 1981, and special needs 2, 92
Education Reform Bill 1988 54
Employment, for language disordered 92
English, teaching of 55
Environment, as cause of language impairment 10
Eurhythmics, Dalcroze 68
Evaluation of child
–first level 46–7
–second level 50
Expression, difficulties in 5, 65, 78

Frith, U. 23–4

Gender, and reading retardation 22
Grammar 12, 13
–abnormal development 15, 16–27, 65
–normal development 15–16
Grauberg, E. 78
Greene, Margaret 90

Haynes, Corinne 8–21
Haynes, & Tempest, B. 15
Hearing loss, conductive 10
Hughes, Martin 77
Hutt, Ella 65–75

ICAN, *see* Invalid Children's Aid Nationwide
Inflection, grammatical 15, 16
Ingram, T.T.S. *et al.* 22
Intervention
–classroom 3, 42, 43–51
first level 44–7
planning 49
second level 47–50
–professional, aims 28
Intonation 14, 15
Invalid Children's Aid Nationwide (ICAN) 81, 91

Kingman Report, 1988 55

Language
–across the curricculum 46, 54–6
–imaginative 46
–oral 42
Language impairment
–estimate of numbers 40–1, 91
–neglect 1–2, 54
–pervasive disorders 4–5, 32
hidden
–specific 3–6, 9, 65
developmental 10
numbers underestimated 2–3, 33
Language unit
–curriculum
growth 71–3
specific elements 69–71
structuring 66–9, 74
–and mainstream classes 66, 69
–population 65–6
–provision 92
–staffing 73–4

Law, J. 43
Learning, active 42, 48
Leicester Polytechnic 31, 36
Length awareness, abnormal 15
Lesser, R. & Hassip, S. 33
Listening, encouraging 45–6
Literacy
–effects of language disorder 3, 5, 15, 52, 56
–pre-literacy skills 46
–in secondary schools 54–6
see also reading; writing
Locke, Ann 2, 40–51

McNeill, D. 8
Materials, teaching 49, 70–2
Mathematics
–assessment of difficulties 78–82
–and language disorder 76, 78–82
–language of 76–7
Memory 5, 16, 88
Methods, teaching, language-dependent 11, 42–3
Mogford, Kay 1–7
Morphology 12, 16
Motor development, and language impairment 4
Movement
–importance in curriculum 67
–Margaret Morris 68
Music, importance in curriculum 67–8

National Child Development Study 32
Nelson, K. 31–2
Noble, Moira 90–6

Observation, school-based 44
Owen, P. & Christie, T. 57

Parents 83–9
–communicative role 45, 85–6
–re-inforcing role 88
–as security provider 86–7
–stimulating and developing role 87–8
–supportive role 85
Passive, acquisition 16
Peter, Laurence 75
Phonology 12, 13–14
–abnormal development 14–15, 19, 22–3, 65
–normal development 14
Pitch awareness, abnormal 15
Play, imaginative, delayed 4
Plurals, irregular 15
Pragmatics 12–14, 14
–abnormal development 20, 65
–normal development 19–20
Profiling, language 11

Reading
–alphabetic stage 23–5, 28
–arrested development 25–8
–difficulties, and speech problems 22, 25, 28
–effect of phonological disorder 15, 22–3, 29
–logographic phase 23, 24, 25–6
–normal development 23–5
–orthographic stage 24
–readiness for 24
–secondary school difficulties 51–3
see also literacy
Reception, language, problems 5, 65, 67, 78
Rehearsal, verbal 16–27
Rhythm, abnormal perception 15, 16
Romaine, S. 19
Rules, language, acquisition 8–9, 15–16
Rutter, M. & Yule, W. 22

SAIL *see* assessments, Staged Assessments in Literacy Project
School
–infant, language in 67
–primary 54
–secondary
literacy in 54–6
literacy problems 51–64
–special 77
Schools Council, 'Language in Use' Programme 54
Screening
–need for in schools 41–2
see also Birmingham, Primary Intervention Procedures; Speech and Language Problems Screening-Test
Self-confidence, encouragement 44–5, 86–7
Self-organisation, encouragement 46
Semantics 11–12, 13–14, 16
–abnormal development 18–19, 20, 65
–normal development 17–18
Senator, Ronald, Musicolour Scheme 68
Signing, in language units 69–70, 80
Skills, alphabetic 28
Skills, social, development 5
Snowling, M. & Stackhouse, J. 26–7

Sound
–blending 23, 26, 28
–segmentation 23, 26, 27–8
Speech and Language Problems Screening-Test (SLPS)
–development and construction 33–8, 93
–need for 31–3
Speech therapy
–and language profiling 11
–provision 91
–and reading disorders 28–9
Spelling
–arrested development 25–8
–difficulties 22–3
–effect of phonological disorder 15, 29
–nonphonetic 25, 26
–normal development 23–5
–phonetic 25–6
–semiphonetic 25–6
–and speech problems 26–7
Stackhouse, Joy 22–30
Steiner, Rudolf, education 68
Strategies
–learning 11, 19–20, 25
–teaching 45–6, 80, 82
Stress, development of 14
Style, shifting 9
Sumner, R. 33
Syntax 12, 14, 16
–abnormal development 19
–five-year-old 8

Teacher
–and knowledge of language 11
–recognition of disorder 33, 41–2
–specialist 2, 91
Teacher training, and language impairment vii, 33, 91, 95
Team management of needs 83
Tense, past 15
Timetabling for special needs 49

Vocabulary
–acquisition 15
–core 70–1
–expansion 17, 46
–variation in development 31–2

Warnock Report, 1978 33
Webster, A. & McConnell, C. 40
Wells, G. 31
Wepman Auditory Discrimination Test 26
Word-finding, difficulties in 65
Writing
–for audience 62
–differentiation of types 57–64, *59–61, 63*
–effect of phonological disorder 15
–organisation 62–3
–and SAIL Project 57–64
–secondary school difficulties 51–64
–use of information 62
see also literacy